The Patient's Encyclopaedia of Urinary Tract Infection
Sexual Cystitis
Interstitial Cystitis

Angela Kilmartin

www.angela.kilmartin.dial.pipex.com

First edition published 2002 by Angela Kilmartin.

Flat 9, 6-9, Bridgewater Square, London EC2Y 8AG.
Website www.angela.kilmartin.dial.pipex.com

Copyright 2002 by Angela Kilmartin

Angela Kilmartin asserts the moral right to be
identified as the author of this work.

ISBN 0-9542627-0-2

This edition
copyright 2004 by Angela Kilmartin

Printed by; Bay Port Press,
645-D Marsat Court,
Chula Vista CA 91911-4649 USA

Distributed by: New Century Press,
1055, Bay Boulevard. Suite C,
Chula Vista CA 91911. USA
Orders: (800) 519-2465
sales@newcenturypress.com

ACKNOWLEDGEMENTS

My life has been bound up with cystitis in one way or another, since my honeymoon in 1966. I have had rare attacks since 1976 but have known the causes. The subject continues to fascinate me and I learn all the time, however, the basic rules are now crystal clear.

It is the dissemination of all this knowledge to sufferers everywhere that still drives me to wreak revenge on cystitis and to inform a still ignorant medical profession. It is my great happiness that they have welcomed my helpful suggestions both to themselves and their patients; they have treated me kindly and I am grateful.

I am also grateful to Paul for years of patience through a miserable early marriage because of my then constant cystitis; to Rowena for so many helpful comments; to Rory for spreading the word at university; to my countless patients for learning opportunities; to countless medical training units for lecture facilities; to many friends who have simply been there for me; to many different publishers at home and abroad; to many secretarial staff over the years; to Bay Port printers, Ron Fraga, Linda and Myra of New Century Press and finally to my great friend Lyn Patterson whose contacts have brought this American edition to fruit.

Angela Kilmartin 2004.

CONTENTS

FORWARD
PREFACE

BOOK ONE - URINARY TRACT INFECTION

PART ONE- BACTERIAL CYSTITIS

FOREWORD

Cystitis is a bane of womankind. From its mildest form of irritation to the severe disease of a life-threatening illness, cystitis has been with us for many centuries. Like other commonly occurring conditions, it has perhaps been put a little to one side by formal medicine; doctors hand out a pocketful of antibiotics and a bit of advice on extra fluids. It was not until Angela Kilmartin started her pioneering work on actually identifying the details of this disease that it came into a medical spotlight.

This book outlines the work she has done for many years to help women with cystitis. It is an excellent account of the background science of the subject and gives very good advice to those who have it. More importantly, perhaps, it advises people on how to prevent cystitis. There is also a very important section on non-bacterial cystitis, for this is a mystery still to some doctors. Angela Kilmartin again dissects the problem and gives first-rate advice on its management. This book is a must for any woman who has ever had the miseries of a urine infection. It is well produced and will help women. I recommend it thoroughly.

Geoffrey Chamberlain, President 1994
Royal College of Obstetricians and Gynaecologists, London.

PREFACE

I lost my honeymoon, all my holidays, my operatic career and my marriage directly or indirectly because of recurrent cystitis. Cystitis is better known in the States as Urinary Tract Infection. It is my avowed aim never to let another woman suffer unnecessarily from such misery and pain.

Every year on 8th August comes the anniversary of my first attack, two days into my honeymoon. I was incontinent, feverish, passing bloody urine, screaming, fainting from the pain and frightened to death. It remains one of my life's most anguished memories.

From then until 1972 I had 78 such attacks, all treated with antibiotics or operations. Thrush from the antibiotics caused equal misery, but nothing was offered to stop the attacks from starting in the first place. I now know for sure that prevention alone is the key to freedom from the pain, misery and stress caused by cystitis.

Unable to guarantee stage appearances, I was forced to abandon a promising career in opera and instead decided to take revenge upon cystitis. In 1971 I founded the U & I Club, (Urinary Infection/You & I) with a magazine specifically for cystitis victims. Unfortunately I had to fold the magazine in 1981 when I went abroad for a long time and the Club has since disbanded. This is the seventh book I have written about cystitis. Many campaigns followed the publication of my first books - a Health Education Council leaflet, a film, TV and radio programmes, a book written for the US market, medical lectures, a video, cystitis action week for Roche Pharmaceuticals and much more.

I have been free of trouble since 1976, when correct prevention routines were finally instituted. To date, millions of other sufferers the world over have been helped or completely cured as a result of my work. I hope this book will help you, too, to be rid once and for all of cystitis.

It is also worth noting here my campaigning work on poisoning from mercury amalgam teeth fillings. Following nearly nine mystifying years mostly bedbound in the late 1980's early 1990's with fifty frightening symptoms, I came to know that I was being poisoned by dental fillings and caps.

Mercury vapour leaches off fillings even more when gold caps are added into the mouth. It is called oral galvanism. Mercury is uptaken in the lungs and stomach where, via blood, it travels to all body tissue, organs and glands causing illness.

Since 1995, following much research and safe removal of a mouthful of fillings, I am well and have published a collection of twenty newsletters from my organisation, Patients Against Mercury Amalgams.

Two campaigns of this magnitude have been burdensome but anger, curiosity and a determination to stop bad practice and bad health have triumphed. The public and professions are better informed and can now prevent all manner of health problems through self help and best practice

Angela Kilmartin 2004

BOOK ONE

Urinary Tract Infection

PART ONE

Bacterial Cystitis

CHAPTER 1

1 Help!

Bacterial cystitis is caused by germs invading the bladder; that is why it is also known as a urinary tract infection. This book will help you to stop it! Say farewell to courses of debilitating antibiotics and their wretched accompaniment, vaginal thrush. You will learn how to prevent, simply, quickly and from today, what could otherwise be a life-long problem with bacterial cystitis.

If you ever visit the ancient site of Hippocrates' teaching hospital founded in 500 BC on the lovely island of Kos, take note of the levels of the hill on which the hospital was built. Each level of the hill (and the hospital) corresponded to a section of the trunk of the human body. The bowels, bladder and genital departments were dug out below the base of the hill into the ground. The very top of the hill was the home of the department of psychiatry. To this day, teaching hospitals put the VD unit either on ground level or below!

Cyst is Greek for a pouch or sac or bladder; *itis* means inflammation which may or may not be caused by infection. About 80 per cent of all cystitis patients have an infection, that is, named bacteria in the urine sample. I had that, too. It was this infection in my urethra and bladder that rocked my young marriage to its core.

For five years I suffered attacks of urinary infection every two to three weeks, and they doubled in misery once permanent vaginal thrush had set in from taking years of antibiotics, knocking the stuffing out of our love and our limits of patient endurance. We barely survived and I believe we used up a mountain of good will, kindness and perseverance fighting my cystitis in those early years, far more than most young marrieds have to face.

Nor did the thrush abate. Nothing was known about how to treat it in the early 1970s except for pessaries and short courses of Nystatin oral tablets (Nystatin is sold as Mycostatin in the US and Australia). There seemed nothing to touch the unremitting candidiasis that had invaded my whole system and kept my vagina sore, red, itchy and full of discharge. Such a vagina could not tolerate sexual intercourse.

So, you see, apart from being very knowledgeable on the help available for sufferers from urinary infections, I know all about the personal social consequences of the suffering. My revenge on it is to write about it and to beat it for you as I did for myself and for the countless women the world over who have followed my advice. Consider this book your first positive step on the road to recovery for good and all. Say farewell to courses of debilitating antibiotics and their wretched accompaniment of vaginal thrush. This book will show you simply and quickly how to prevent, *from today*, what could be a life-long problem with bacterial cystitis.

The kind of help that I offer for sufferers from urinary infections is *preventive* help. How much sooner would you rather prevent the dreaded twinges that signal the onset of yet another attack? Of course, this book also includes first aid for helping to get rid of an attack, but that, to my way of thinking, spells failure; failure to stop that attack from ever having started in the first place. It is much more clever to prevent it and to prevent it for good.

Stopping attacks has very beneficial effects all round:

1. You do not need to take further courses of antibiotics.
2. You save a huge amount of money by not having to buy these antibiotics.
3. Trips to the doctor for the condition may cease altogether: no more agonies in the waiting room or difficulties in getting to the surgery.
4. Long-term trouble for the immune system is halted.
5. No further risks of vaginal thrush or candidiasis.
6. Intercourse can be safely and happily enjoyed.
7. Your partner can no longer use this excuse to 'stray'.
8. You can go to work regularly - not have a week off every time you suffer an attack.
9. You can guarantee to do the weekly shopping trip.
10. Fear of future attacks disappears altogether.

Take it from me, preventing trouble is not only easy and cheap, it is also pure bliss to be free of the symptoms.

Symptoms

The classic symptoms of urinary infection are:

- pain when you pass urine
- frequency of urination and the urgent need to go
- bleeding from the urethral tube as you pass urine
- backache

- fever or raised temperature
- smelly urine

These symptoms present in variable forms. The pain, for instance, starts as a shivery twinge as you finish passing urine on a seemingly ordinary visit to the toilet. That shivery twinge sends a cold, upward ripple of sensation in the urethral tube. If steps to abort it are not taken straight away, these twinges progress quite quickly to scalding, pain, and further on to what I always describe as the 'scalpel' stage. 'Broken glass' is another common description of the intensely sharp and excruciating pain that accompanies the advanced stage of infection.

Now let's look at a few of these symptoms in more detail.

Frequency and Urgency

Do I know about this! In my early attacks I sometimes did not 'make it' to the toilet. When this urgency strikes there is absolutely no question of 'holding it': that urine has a will of its own and you leave the close vicinity of a bathroom at your peril! The very delicate mechanisms of bladder and urethral action are thrown into top gear in a desperate attempt to flush the invading bacteria out. It is a defence system that becomes automatic once the invasion signals are sent out.

It works the same way if a food or drink has an allergic effect, or if a chemical upsets the sensitive vulval skin. These non-bacterial causes are discussed in later chapters.

Bleeding

This is a particularly horrible symptom, and a definite sign that a severe bacterial invasion is infiltrating the urethral and bladder lining. It happens quickly in women who have had many past attacks and who now bear scars inside their urethra and bladder. These minute scars are weaker than fresh skin and have a diminished ability to repel bacteria. The more scars you acquire, the more likely you will bleed. Once bacteria gain entrance to the bloodstream, *backache* and *fever* will start. You will feel very ill and may start to shake as your kidneys become infected.

This is really dangerous. Too much of this may scar your kidneys for life, they may become disfigured and lose their smoothness and bean-like shape. The next step could be to lose the use of these two vital organs. Dialysis twice a week would keep you alive but at great cost and with a severe reduction in the quality of life.

In the USA, there is little knowledge at all on self help and so much surgery has been done on women's bladders that they no longer function and, after years of repeated infections and dilations, the trouble is so chronic that they sometimes need removing. Interstitial Cystitis has its own section in this Encyclopaedia and I will not dwell on it here, except to add that laboratory work and doctors between them are failing to diagnose correctly.

Although I have had one book out in the US since 1979, I am not there in person to do publicity and no self-help really exists. The result is that American women have gone from bad to worse by the million. Fear of litigation keeps urologists talking about this 'new' condition, IC, and prevents the truth from emerging.

We in Britain have not had a similar proliferation (in part because I am here to stop it!) but increasingly ignorant urologists are encouraging patients to think in terms of IC to mask medical inability and ignorance.

There is much to be gained from stopping early attacks on the first twinges. You absolutely must protect your kidneys because you cannot grow new ones and prevention saves you from most of the misery of the ordinary attack and from a lot of unnecessary expense as well.

Anyone with an ulcerated bladder lining might like to insist that urine samples are cultured for Myco bacteria which may be responsible for chronic pain and bladder ulceration. Only one antibiotic works against them.

If antibiotics ever seem to increase bladder pain this may point to a fungal infestation in which case anti-fungal systemic drugs like Sporanox or Itraconazole should be prescribed for at least two weeks. If there is some small improvement continue anti-fungal systemic treatment. Bladder urine and biopsies can be tested for Candida if the laboratory is so requested.

Dental links

In 1923 a Dr. Weston Price in Cleveland, Ohio, USA was heavily involved in proving that accepted knowledge of dental treatments was unjustifiable given his profound experiments on rabbits and the thousands of Case Histories that came his way. The two massive volumes into which he collated his thousands of experiments are called:

Volume I - Dental Infections Oral and Systemic Disease. Volume II - Dental Infections and the Degenerative Diseases.

They are available to dentists from the British Dental Association Library in

Wimpole Street, London. The general public may make an appointment to go and view them but the books may not be taken out except by a dentist registered at the BDA. Reprints may also be bought from America via a Mastercard for 180 dollars from The Price Pottinger Foundation, telephone 001-619-574-7763.

In these volumes are to be found causes of every manner of systemic diseases originating in teeth. There are scores of pages on kidney disease caused by bad teeth and bad dental treatments, in particular Root Canal Therapy which Dr. Price asserts, backed up by his experiments, causes this. In one big chapter on kidneys, apart from the huge number of mentions elsewhere, there are two pages on bladder troubles.

Both men and women as victims of dentally focused bladder troubles are dealt with in this exciting section. Chronic cystitis, i.e. long-term pain, infection and frequency may, he claims, be caused by poor dental treatment and jaw infections. He discloses ulcerated bladders in rabbits which had previously been implanted with diseased root-canalled teeth from both men and women who have had some kind of central nervous system disturbance. In so-called Interstitial Cystitis, bladder ulcers appear to be regularly found. Unrelieved pain which may indeed emanate from an involvement with the spinal cord might be relieved if the source is looked for in the spinal column or jaws somewhere. That ulcers are the key link may not be coincidental but simply the bladder reflecting the state of jaw ulceration as well.

Those searching for an answer might also look back to your own diaries showing any root canal treatment. Systemic reactions in any gland or organ can commence thereafter at any interval. This may become immediately obvious or some months or years later. No-one would be thinking of linking the teeth to the bladder! But it's worth a ponder and Dr. Price is quite specific in his books.

Root Canal Infection

Root canal treatment causes long-term chronic infective processes to invade jaw tissue and on into lymph/ nerve/blood pathways. It could be worth removing the root canal treatment if diary dates coincide with bladder troubles, by full tooth extraction and monitoring the result. Allow time for bladder ulcers to deplete after any tooth or canal extraction though usually systemic disease or pain elsewhere other than the bladder can resolve exceptionally fast after extraction. Some people literally throw away their crutches on the journey home from the extraction!

Root Canal Treatments promote infection in the dentine tubules and until the colony of bacteria increases or the toxins start to leak into the canal itself, the patient will not become aware. Bacteria are usually Staphylococcus as Dr. Price showed but the jaw infections spreading outwards from infected root canal treatments or careless extractions can show mixed anaerobes and aerobes. These will necessitate very heavy courses of mixed antibiotics to control the infection. It is always worth organising samples from these extractions and curettings of jawbone and tissue in case antibiotics and proof are required. Then sensitive antibiotics can be specifically prescribed.

If this is not the cause of the ulceration then it might be Mycobacteria (see the Interstitial Cystitis book) or even fungi. There is also a group of bacteria known as Bacters that can be found in the bladder if the laboratory is sufficiently sophisticated and able. Citrobacter is one member of this group more commonly found in reputable labs. Such unusual bacteria may not be tested for in most laboratories, so ask and show this section to the relevant doctors, also determine whether your local lab has a facility to test for these infections.

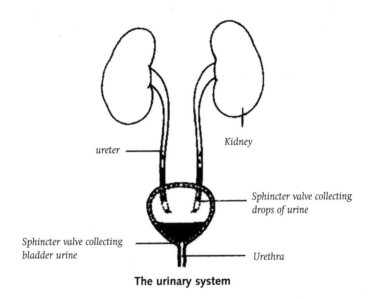

ureter

Kidney

Sphincter valve collecting drops of urine

Sphincter valve collecting bladder urine

Urethra

The urinary system

The urinary system

Kidneys sift waste body products into liquid and send it down each ureter as urine, until the gentle pressure of several drops on the sphincter valves influences them to open up and allow the urine into the bladder. I have watched this happening during a procedure called a *cystoscopy*, which I was once allowed to view, with the help of a microscope in the *cystoscope* which is an instrument with a light for viewing the urethra and bladder. I was thrilled to see this clever little internal activity. It goes on 24 hours a day for as long as you live!

When sufficient urine has collected in the bladder the urethral sphincter bows to pressure and signals to you to go to the toilet, where you then let it all flow out.

When the urethra is invaded by bacteria, this invasion progresses as shown below:

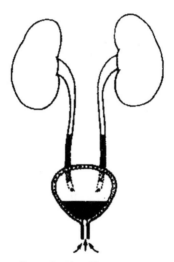

External perianal bacteria rising
throughout urinary system then
into bloodstream

The urethra invaded by bacteria

This first chapter is called Help ! You can already see that there is a lot of it, so cheer up!

CHAPTER TWO

2 Don't Cry!

Curse and swear, yes! But crying usually renders you incapable of any action. Being blinded by tears means you cannot walk round, you cannot get busy to help yourself and it demoralizes you still more. You hunch up over a hankie and feel utterly desperate, as though you have been hit on the head with a brick. Not another one! 'What will Ricky think when he gets home and finds me like this again! I can't take any more time off work!', or 'Where can I send the children for the day?', or 'I can't get to the doctor before tonight even if I will be well enough by then; Mom's out for the day so she can't help. I just feel so hopeless, so depressed, the pain's getting worse and I'll finish up sitting on the toilet all day.'

The tears pour down, you need another hankie and you start to feel feverish. Every time you pass miserably small amounts of scalding urine, you shiver and yell and cry some more. Then the fear starts, and maybe the bleeding if you have had lots of attacks before. After an hour or so you cannot walk easily, so down onto the carpet you sink, still crying in waves of panic and self-pity. 'Why me?!'

I have been there, reader, I have been there many times and so have countless others. You, nowadays, are relatively lucky, though. You have this book to read; there was absolutely nothing written or suggested for patients before 1972, when I first started my work and wrote my first articles, after years of suffering with cystitis.

Stop crying - get angry instead. Build up your anger and have a good swear. Once you are up on your feet, go to the kitchen and get busy. Mentally adjust the anger now to productive activity and a wish to fight this rising, intrusive pain and embarrassing frequency. Think yourself lucky it has started at home, that you are not on the bus or the train, or stuck in a traffic jam somewhere!

Think yourself lucky that, as you progress through this book you will learn how to prevent further days like today. Do not give in to it, not now you are going to arm yourself with the best help in the world. It is help that works perfectly and will make such days a thing of the past. Do stop crying, you are going to feel much better in an hour or so!

Practical Steps

What sequence of practical steps should you take when an attack of cystitis begins? Whenever it starts, no matter what time of day or night, TAKE A URINE SAMPLE BEFORE YOU DO ANY DRINKING.

How to Take a Mid-stream Urine Sample (MSU)
1. Pour boiling water from a kettle into a 1pint (20 fl. oz/500 ml) heat-proof measuring jug to sterilize it. Just shake it dry and then cover it with a clean cloth until you need it.
2. By the same method, sterilize a small glass jar and lid, if you do not already have a sterile jar from the doctor or pharmacy.
3. Take both to the bathroom and set them down.
4. Still standing up, take two or three wet cotton balls and clean your urethral and vaginal openings.
5. Clean the rim of the toilet bowl, then sit on this, rather than the seat, so that it is easier to pass the pyrex jug beneath you.
6. Pass a little urine into the toilet, then catch the midstream in the pyrex jug.
7. Finish the stream into the pan.
8. Clean up, pour the urine sample from the jug into the jar, seal it with the lid.
9. Label the jar with your name, address, the time and your doctor's name.
10. Store this in the fridge for the time being - but get it to the doctor or laboratory quickly.

This is obviously easy to do at home, but if an attack starts when you are at work or out, try to get home, if you are on holiday, get to your hotel bedroom and get that specimen organized. It should go very quickly to a laboratory via your doctor or a special clinic or a helpful friend. If it has to wait a bit, it must be put straight in the fridge.

Go to the doctor if you want and get some antibiotics 'in case', but you may not need to take them.

Once you reach home, or your hotel or, of course, at work if you know that you will not be able to make it home in time, proceed as recommended in the sections that follow.

Three Hour First-Aid Management Procedure
Having already taken the MSU,
1. Drink half a pint (10 fl. oz/250 ml) of water straight away and another half pint every 20 minutes for three hours. No more and no less. If you drink before

taking the MSU, the sample will be too diluted to analyse correctly.

2. In that initial half-pint (and repeating on the second and third hour), mix any of the following:
   - 1 level teaspoon of bicarbonate of soda or
   - potassium citrate or something similar in USA from any pharmacy to alkalinise urine. Follow packet instructions.
3. Take three strong painkillers (such as paracetamol or Tyelenol) with another quick glass of water, and a further dose in three hours' time.
4. Fill two hot-water bottles, if you have them. Sit in a comfy chair or go to bed and wedge one bottle at your back, cover the other with a towel and wedge that up between your legs over your vulva.
5. Help the bladder to flush even more by taking a diuretic such as Frusemide, if your doctor will allow you, or by having one strong cup of *coffee* on the hour every hour for just three hours. Water, anyway, is a good diuretic.

This simple first aid has many advantages:

- You will protect your kidneys from permanent scarring.
- The pain is very swiftly reduced.
- Any bleeding will shortly stop.
- By acting fast, bacterial growth rate is halted.
- You can stay at work if you must.
- There may prove to be no necessity for antibiotics at all.
- It is very cheap!

Once the three hours are up you will be much better. Do not attempt to change the timing or the dosages; they have been carefully worked out. For instance, extra water will alter your blood pressure and you may feel dizzy, but with the half-pint every 20 minutes for three hours you should not have any adverse reaction.

The bicarbonate and potassium citrate act to alkalanize urine so that bacteria, whose preferred environment is mild acidity, cannot thrive. Choose whichever one you like. You are most likely to have some bicarbonate in the house but getting others will probably mean a trip to the local pharmacy.

If you hate the bicarbonate in water, try it in a small amount of jam followed by a drink.

After the three hours, keep a half-pint going down about every hour, and tail that off as the situation stabilizes. Painkillers are also very useful in calming bladder nerve endings and stopping them from unnecessary activity once the bacteria begin to go.

Washing the Perineum (Area Between the Legs)

A lot of women ask me whether it is helpful to do any perineal washing during an attack. At this first-aid stage, without the urine sample result, you do not know whether this attack is due to bacterial invasion or something else.

(For this section of the book, dealing solely with infection, I am going to assume that the attack being dealt with is caused by bacterial infection, so I will suggest the following washing. You should understand, though, as you progress through the book, that recurrent urinary infections will soon be a thing of the past because you will learn how to prevent them. I have, therefore, put this first aid early in the book because it may be the last time you need it!)

If we do assume for this once that, in view of previous attacks which have shown positive bacteria in the urine sample, this attack is probably also due to bacteria, then we may also assume that your whole perineum is, at this moment, running with bacteria. So how to clean it thoroughly?

Whilst sitting on the toilet, pour some warm water from a bottle down the front over the vulva to wash urinary bacteria off the skin. Then pat dry with a clean wash-cloth or even kitchen roll just for now. The use of kitchen roll is only for very temporary situations; **never** use toilet paper or tissues to dry the perineum after washing, since small pieces of tissue break off and get left to gather bacteria on the skin. Obviously using paper is required after passing a stool or if used briefly for dabbing dry after passing urine.

When You Have the Urine Sample Results

Once the results are back, you have more evidence with which to pursue further detective work. The next chapter has more details about this.

Supposing it is positive yet again? Not to worry: your troubles are over because following the advice in this book will stop further attacks. If the result shows a heavy growth and the condition is still unstable (that is, you are still feeling lots of twinges), then appropriately sensitive antibiotics should be taken. Three to five days should be enough. Continued sensible drinking, painkillers and urinary voiding will give you comfort and keep decreasing the bacterial growth

Conventional Medical Help

The chances are that you have picked up this book because you haven't got anywhere with the medical profession's help, so it will cheer you up to know that a report from the Institute of Urology in the UK states that patient hygiene came out top in a survey of what prevents cystitis attacks in young women. Sadly, the doctors involved did not bother to get the Report published but they were delighted with the results.

If you haven't tried self-help you will have been subjected to medical 'help'. This currently comprises:

- *Urine samples*
  Mid-stream Urine MSU
- *Antibiotics*
  Prescribed whether the MSU is positive or negative
- *Intra -Venous Pyelogram – IVP. Scan.*
  An X-ray of the kidneys and bladder, or a scan.
- *Cystoscopy*
  The surgeon looks up a cystoscope into the bladder
- *Dilation*
  Widening or enlarging the urethra or bladder
- *Cauterization*
  Burning away infected and scarred urethral or bladder skin
- *Urodynamics*
  Checking the working of the urinary system
- *Micturating cystogram*
  Measuring the urinary flow

There are various operations to suit particular results of investigations, such as 'bladder washouts', or surgery to correct a prolapsed bladder or to remove stones or obstructions. One good IVP should show whether further urological work is necessary. Do not submit to the surgeon at all if your bladder has behaved perfectly normally until a given incident or time. Look into the particular causes of your infection and try self-help treatments before 'going medical'.

If you find Cranberry Juice helps, I have no quarrel, but I call this a treatment. It is costly, it can cause bladder thrush/Candida from fruit sugars; it's a publicity gimmick, it's something else to lug home and it doesn't work for most people. Germs respond to being washed off like surgeons do before operating. Surgeons do not drink Cranberry juice, they wash! Men and women unfortunate enough to have had a colostomy (bladder removal) are permanently prone to kidney and bladder infections. Their hygiene has to be superb but even this may be insufficient because of the internal links with bowel tissue. Cranberry has been known to provide an added support in these cases.

Who Gets Cystitis?

Research shows the largest group of victims to be aged 18 to 35 years, but little girls and older women also get it for various reasons. Women who are pregnant form quite a well-known group of bacterial sufferers, and labour can set off a urinary infection. Infections frequently begin during a stay in hospital. In fact, over 30 per cent of all infections contracted in hospital are urinary infections.

Some women never get it, and I am often asked my thoughts on this. There are certain factors that can determine whether a woman will be predisposed to this type of infection:

1. The nearness of the anal opening to the urethral tube varies from woman to woman. Some women may have a lengthy gap, while others may have a shorter gap allowing easier bacterial access to the urethral opening.

2. Some women still wipe 'back to front' when they go to the toilet, enabling germs to enter the urethra easily.

3. Some women may not have a strong enough resistance to the bacteria.

4. Daughters often 'copy' parental hygiene procedures, rightly or wrongly.

5. Failing to pass urine regularly allows germs a longer time to penetrate the urethra and set up a small colony.

6. Some women automatically wash before sex, helping to ensure that germs do not spread from their anal passage to their vagina.

7. Some women shower or bathe after a bowel movement as part of their automatic daily routine and avoid bacterial travel.

8. Constipation plays its part, too. There is a big bacterial build-up in large, unpassed feces. When they are eventually passed there may be a stronger bacterial presence on the anal opening. Many women are frequently constipated, especially before a period. Diarrhoea or loose stools also leave residue.

Hygiene in all cases prevents this bacterial travel.

CHAPTER 3

3 Get Some Answers!

You have never asked for the result of a urine sample? Shame on you. It is your sample, not the doctor's. Not only do you have a right to ask what is in it, you absolutely must. It is the biggest clue to enable you to start work on the cause or causes of your cystitis.

A positive MSU (mid-stream urine) sample means that infection is present. It will say:

Heavy Growth
Medium Growth
Insignificant Growth
No Growth

The layout of laboratory forms can vary and appear technical. When counselling women, I take account of the following as well as the words:

- Any ++ signs against red, white or epithelial cell reports mean inflammation or infection is present.
- Whether the woman drank water before taking the sample, which would dilute it.
- Whether antibiotics have been taken in the past 3 weeks.
- Whether symptoms declined if sympathy antibiotics were taken during previous attacks. Antibiotics only work against infection, nothing else.

False results often occur if these factors influenced the sample. I used to think it a good idea to take a 'clearance MSU' after a course of antibiotics. Of course, this would be negative because antibiotics continue their influence for several weeks against a particular bacterium. But other bacteria from the bowel may start a new bladder infection if not prevented. Therefore I now disagree with taking clearance MSU's, because they can be misleading.

The laboratory must also tell the doctor to which antibiotic group the bacterium is sensitive. A rational choice can then be made, taking into account a variety of factors including the age of the patient, whether she is pregnant or not, etc. If the result says 'mixed growth', domination of the infection by stronger bacteria within it may occur. The first antibiotic may need to be replaced by one sensitive to the dominant bacteria. Only three days need to pass to establish that antibiotics need replacing.

Three full days of any antibiotic is sufficient to tell you whether it has defeated the bacteria. If twingeing rises on the second, third or fourth day, ring the doctor and ask whether the sensitivity culture shows other bacteria or whether there are further antibiotic choices for this bacteria.

You must know the correct sequence of events at this time:

1. Collect the sample under proper conditions.
2. Make sure it arrives in the laboratory during working hours.
3. Make sure there is a full bacterial AND sensitivity culture.
4. Do the three hour management process AFTER the sample has been taken.
5. If it is certainly an infection (i.e. you had neglected hygiene rules) take prescribed antibiotics.
6. If these fail after three days, ring the doctor.
7. Requesting a second urine sample may prove unhelpful since you will have drunk a lot and diluted the bacteria. Also, the first antibiotics may still affect the second sample, giving a false result.
8. It pays to take the first urine sample very seriously.

By the time you get the result, you will have had three days of monitoring your own condition which will help you to decide whether or not to take the recommended drug. Generally, I think that any feeling of discomfort, soreness or twingeing, or swollen and red perineum at this time, should be dealt with by a short course of antibiotics. If vaginal thrush has presented itself on earlier occasions when taking a course of antibiotics, then your doctor should prescribe a 10-day course of Nystatin (known in the US and Australia as Mycostatin) oral tablets together with the best vaginal pessaries. Sporanox or Diflucan (anti-fungal oral treatments) will help just as well.

Just using vaginal pessaries does nothing to treat the intestinal candida upsurge and so, even after completing the pessary course, vaginal thrush may return. Oral treatment helps prevent this.

Women who cannot tolerate antibiotics should benefit greatly by the first-aid methods advocated in Chapter 1; daily prevention is important for all women but even more so for them.

Special Clinics

If you do have a sore, swollen or reddened perineum (lie on the bed with a mirror and look.), go to the Emergency Room or ask whether there is a Sexual health/ Genito-urinary unit taking 'walk-in' patients in your area.

When you are seen you may be asked whether you have any 'waterworks' trouble as well. Why they can't just say 'urinary symptoms' I can't imagine! 'Waterworks' means sewage and water supply to me!

They will take a urine sample, a vaginal and cervical swab. Swabs are taken painlessly by inserting long cotton wool buds and not only do samples get looked at immediately, but a full three day culture in the laboratory is also done. A cervical smear is not the same as a cervical swab. The smear tests only for cancer, the swab tests for bacteria. If something is found when they put the specimen under the microscope, you will go home with appropriate treatment according to the condition diagnosed.

Should you be told that there is no infection in the urine or on the swabs in the special clinic, this does not mean that you are 'imagining' your symptoms. It can mean that what is present is not a recognizable sexually transmitted disease. Some of these clinics stick very strictly to reporting only on venereal or sexually transmitted diseases. They do not seem inclined to bend the rules in order to be efficient. It makes no monetary sense to take this attitude and compel the poor patient to use the resources of another department as well. She would have to revisit her doctor, get a referral and wait for an appointment in the gynaecology or urology unit.

Not all special clinics take this strict attitude, and because most women seem, even these days, to have to pluck up some courage to visit one, the doctors mostly do their best to re-assure and to examine gently. Such clinics provide an excellent service - and a free one, if you live in the UK and go to an NHS (National Health Service) clinic. I have used them myself. It is all very good value and you will be seen very quickly. Of course, your family doctor can also take swabs which go on the delivery van mid-morning to the nearest hospital laboratory.

Another good reason to use such medical facilities is to double check the results reported by the hospital laboratory to which your doctor sent your sample. There are many reasons why your original sample may result in an *inaccurate* diagnosis:

- You may have forgotten to refrigerate it at home.
- Once at the doctor's surgery (office) it may again not be refrigerated.
- The collection van may be early, late or not come at all that day, which leaves

your sample hanging around.
- It may be a Friday without a late van delivery to the laboratory, so that your sample is not seen until after the weekend!
- You yourself may have taken an unclean specimen.
- Drinking *before* taking the sample dilutes the numbers of bacteria.
- Antibiotics taken for anything within the past three weeks can make the sample negative.

Any or all of these factors could give an inaccurate result. Only on your local laboratory's past record can you be reasonably certain of how efficient it is, for instance, if *all* your past vaginal swabs have shown positive something or other, or if all your past urine samples have shown positive bacterial counts. By the same token, if they have all shown negative results, in either instance you should use the resources of the special clinic to do a double-check. Or you might want to go to a private specialist to get a second opinion. Ask where the samples are sent, though: if it is the *same* laboratory then you may be wasting your money.

A Positive Sample

So, the urine sample is positive. It is not enough just to know that much. You must ask what the bacterium is called and where it comes from. Most urinary infections are caused by:

- **Escherichia coliform**
- **Streptococcus fecalis**

then, less commonly, by

- Staphylococcus
- Klebsiella
- Proteus
- Pseudomonas

Pseudomonas is not normal bowel flora, it overgrows like candida if you are given antibiotics. (There is more about all these bacteria in the next chapter.)

These organisms cohabit in the intestines and bowel of every human being. *This means that the infection in your urine sample is due to your own bacteria, which has come from your body, no one else's!* This is the most important factor to know when trying to sort yourself out. No doctor ever explains this. In short, you are causing your own urinary infection! Eighty per cent of you, all reading this book because you are suffering from urinary **infections**, are causing your own misery! (Once again I must stress that this applies to women with a proven, named infection in their urine specimens. There are countless other reasons for negative urine samples where the symptoms of cystitis appear the same but the cause or causes have nothing to do with real bacterial infection).

The Truth about Toilet Seats

Toilet seats can be contaminated. Even if not from a direct vulvo/pubic contact, the act of flushing propels bacteria in water spray some six yards up and out from the bowl. This has been studied and written up! Coliforms have been found six feet away! Most women hate unknown toilets and will either not sit down or will line the seat with tissue paper. (By the way, never hover! It stops the bladder emptying completely because you are too tense.) If you need to pass a stool in a place other than home, line the seat with toilet roll paper before you sit down. It is the front part of the seat which is potentially the most bacterially contaminated, but it does depend on the place, whether children or old people use it and how often it is cleaned. Perhaps the back part of the seat and the bowl itself look wet? Dry it up and then put paper at the back of the seat so you can sit comfortably. Bacteria can pass through moistened soft paper and then transfer practically anywhere, which is why cleaning the toilet and washing your hands afterwards are so important.

Passing urine in a strange toilet isn't that tricky. I find that a couple of sheets of paper placed slightly to right of centre allow me to sit on my right side, relaxed enough to empty the bladder fully. The difficulty really comes when there is no paper! Then what? Try one handbag tissue instead. Men don't know how lucky they are!

Always wash your hands afterwards. I do wish that elbow operated taps and soap dispensers were available in public toilets, as they are in operating theatres for the surgeons. I hate touching all those taps and soaps and drying facilities with my hands or fingertips; I never really feel clean until I am in my own hotel room or my bathroom at home.

If you are out and in charge of a little girl who wants to go the toilet, you must line the front of the seat and help support her while she goes. When my daughter first began using the toilet, I always squatted in front of her and held her under her armpits and around her rib cage. It is so important for such tiny bladders to empty completely and expel any germs around the vulval area, little girls do tend to want to 'hold it'! They should be told not to, and taught clearly from early years of the dangers of retaining 'nasty germs inside that may start to hurt you'.

If she wants to pass a stool, stay with her and teach her time and again until you are sure she knows no other way than to wipe around her back passage from behind. Wiping the back passage *from behind* and not touching the front is an enormous aid to preventing urinary infection in little girls.

Teach also about lining the seat when they use a toilet away from home, so that a dirty school toilet doesn't psychologically prevent them from going when they need to.

As a little girl sits on the seat, even if it is lined, she will still want to use her hands on the sides to help support herself. This is unavoidable. Before sitting, she should be taught to break off and hold two or three sheets of paper with which, later, to dab her vulval area dry and then, of course, to wash her hands properly at the basin after pulling the flush.

She should also be shown to put in the basin plug so that hot and cold water can mix to a comfortable temperature for washing her hands. Plenty of soap and rinsing well are good habits to adopt.

Some of you may think this is all very obvious, but would be surprised at how many mothers do not take the time and trouble to get these simple messages across to their daughters. Some years ago, the mother of a five-year-old girl contacted me. Her daughter had constant, proven urinary infections and lived on antibiotics, though scans and examinations all proved negative. When I questioned her, she told me she was only bathing this child once a week.' I was patient and practical. The child must be bathed daily. Recently I had cause to ring her, only to find that the now eight-year-old girl is frequently hospitalized, her life painful and still disrupted with infections.

'You are bathing her daily as I said?'

'Well, not really, we're busy and I forget, I suppose it's my fault really, she baths every three or four days.'

I was almost speechless with rage and told her so in great fury. Why hadn't the doctors asked about hygiene habits and, upon being told, refused to treat her daughter until the daily bath was in place? This constitutes neglect, I think, on the mother's part.

I can't bear not to say a word about small boys here! It is not so much for their sake that I do as for the sake of their future girlfriends and wives. My son was circumcised at three days old. His penis does not harbour infectious material under a non-existant foreskin! I also took just as much trouble over my son's toileting habits as my daughter's. This extends even to basin tidiness and to cleaning round the bath for the next person.

At aged eight my son was taught to clean a toilet correctly. If my children left any kind of unacceptable mess in bathrooms, they were told instantly to come and wipe up.

I have been asked many times during counselling sessions how best to clean a toilet. Here's the best method;

1. Keep cream cleaner and a heavy string cloth on a peg in the bathroom. Also a good brush-cleaning set.
2. Lift the seat and squirt some cream cleaner around the bowl. Scrub the bowl all round with the long-handled toilet brush.
3. Flush and scrub again, finally rinsing the brush under the last fresh water flowing into the bowl.
4. Now wet the string cloth under the hot tap and squirt a few drops of cream cleaner onto it.
5. Clean the topside of the seat first, then the underside and lastly the rim of the porcelain bowl.
6. Open out the cloth and thoroughly rinse it in hot water.
7. Now wipe the cream cleaner off the porcelain rim, then the underside of the seat. Rinse the cloth again.
8. Repeat item 7 and then wipe the cream cleaner off the topside of the seat.
9. Rinse the open cloth (don't scrunch it into a ball) thoroughly under hot running water.
10. Now wipe that topside of the seat once more.
11. Rinse the cloth well for a final time, squeeze it and leave it hanging exposed to air and well ventilated.

You notice that I haven't mentioned disinfectants at all. I don't believe they are necessary in the first place and, in the second, disinfectant on the seat itself can cause horrible skin troubles (it is not a problem in the pan unless 'splashback' happens when a stool is passed). I have specifically mentioned using a cream cleaner because you can see traces of it if you haven't thoroughly wiped it off. It is this kind of cleaner that I use at home and I find it meets my own (very stringent!) standards.

Trichomonas

Trichomonas is worth mentioning here. It causes a nasty vaginal discharge and you can get a vicious dose of cystitis or urethritis from it. Trichomonas is a water-borne parasite which lives in pan water. If your toilet pan is quite deep and the water splashes back onto your bottom when you pass a stool, the trichomonal parasite can splash onto your skin. Wiping it with toilet paper won't work. The parasite quickly swims in vulval moisture, starts to breed and can be sexually transmitted.

Trichomonas dies in air and lives in moisture. Stop the 'splash-back' by placing a sheet of toilet paper on the surface of the water in the pan before passing a stool.

The more people using a toilet, the more it needs cleaning. Flat- or house-shares involving several young people require a lot of cleaning. If you have been getting urinary infections regularly, keep the cream cleaner and cloth in your own room and clean that toilet before you personally use it. When cleaned, just dab the seat dry with some toilet paper before you sit on it, so that you can happily discount the seat as the remotest source of infection and so that you can do the essential bottle-washing (described in Chapter 5).

What Happens to Your Urine Sample?

Returning to swabs and urine samples, the one and only request that I make prior to a counselling appointment is; 'please ring your doctor and ask for photocopies of the results of swabs and MSUs to bring with you.' I used to be satisfied with verbal reports, but no longer.

It is absolutely extraordinary that so many victims of urinary infection don't know what is in their urine sample results.

When you take your sample it needs to be collected carefully, as I have said. If you and your doctor are working well together you should be allowed two or three spare sterile sample jars with labels so that you can take a specimen early, if a new attack starts.

When your urine sample arrives at a hospital laboratory, having been personally delivered or taken by the collecting van which picks them up from the doctor, it is checked in, much like a guest arriving at a hotel reception!

Although out-patients' urine samples do not arrive till mid morning, the laboratory is already at work, if it is within a large hospital, checking in samples from the various wards. A steady number of hospital porters and orderlies comes to the reception desk with bundles of samples of all sorts from all over the hospital and the local health authority catchment area. Some days can be busy - for instance on days when local ante-natal clinics are held and routine samples sent off to the hospital laboratory.

The laboratory usually works six days a week, but emergency work will be done on a Sunday! In the laboratory where I followed the processing of urine samples, they have their own in house procedures or protocol. All hospitals are free to make their own protocol, but every laboratory is subjected to regular spot-checks by a special central public health laboratory.

At the reception desk, two sorters separate sample jars, which should be (but are not always) clearly labelled, from their forms upon which the doctor has stated a request for analysis together with the patient's details.

The details from the doctor are *instantly*, right there at the reception desk, computerized and the specimen given a number on the screen. The computer details are then printed out onto a sticker which is stuck on the back of the original form. All these forms are taken through to the offices of the various microbiologists, who then decide which samples should be looked at under a microscope in addition to the culturing overnight which *all* samples undergo.

All urine samples from urology offices or from the urological ward within the general hospital - are automatically sent for microscopy (put under the microscope) as well as cultured. Any others are judged by sight if they are cloudy with pus and blood or clear, and then added on to the others indicated for microscopy. For some specific clinical indications it is useful to look for pus cells or peculiar red cells. The microbiologist is very dependent on having the form filled in properly.

Computer No.	*001*
Patient's No.	*45*
Patient's name, birth date, sex	*Bloggs, 28/11/41,Female*
Consultant's Name	*Mr. Waterflow*
Location	*General Hospital, Looe*
Doctor	*L. Bol, MD*
Specimen No.	*287 (written on lid of jar)*
Investigation type	*MSU culture and sensitivity*
Antibiotics	*none taken recently*
Diagnosis?	*Urinary infection*

The computer has an individual number for each patient and for each specimen, which is distinct from the specimen's new number freshly inked on the lid of the specimen jar.

While the forms are with the microbiologists in their offices, the actual urine specimens mount up quickly enough into a tray-load. This tray is taken to the 'urine bench'. Other testing benches are for respiratory, gynaecological, wounds, fecal, leukaemic and neonatal specimens. HIV (AIDS) patients' specimens have their own bench in a separate room.

On the urine bench the tray-load is placed onto a 'cold table' which is refrigerated to keep the specimens in a good state until they are ready to be 'plated', i.e. when small amounts of urine are put onto a special culture dish or plate.

A medical laboratory scientific officer - MLSO for short - is now in charge of the specimens. One may set up as few as 250 specimens a day on culture plates or far more than that. Double-checking the specimen number against culture plate number is of prime importance. Let's follow Rita Bloggs' specimen:

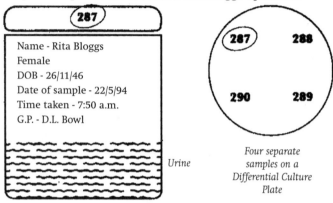

Name - Rita Bloggs
Female
DOB - 26/11/46
Date of sample - 22/5/94
Time taken - 7:50 a.m.
G.P. - D.L. Bowl

Urine

Four separate samples on a Differential Culture Plate

**Urinary sample form;
four separate samples on a differential quarter culture plate**

The MLSO writes up a batch of numbers on the differential culture plates - four numbers per plate. Differential culture (also called culture quarter) plates are thin, clear round plastic holders with tops. The numbers go clockwise in quarters and mistakes are seldom made.

The MLSO then prepares to put a droplet of Rita's urine into the quarter of the plate containing her number. The plate has a green/agar/protein film (green = dye; agar = seaweed protein; other proteins and carbohydrates = bacterial food source) upon which most of the possible organisms in Rita's urine will grow. The shaken urine jar is placed on a green paper towel so that any spillage gets absorbed. In sterile packaging on the bench are thin *bacterial loops*. Each loop is a long, fine plastic stick which, when the end is dipped in the urine, retains just one precise microlitre. This microlitre of urine (droplet) is smeared onto Rita's section of the quarter culture plate.

The object of the culture is to give a rough idea of how many organisms are grown on the plate overnight. Several other methods may be used, but laboratories usually end up doing the simplest thing because there are so many specimens to process.

A positive MSU is technically one where there are more than 10,000 organisms of a single type present in one millilitre of urine. If the MSU was not taken cleanly by the patient, or if the specimen has hung around for a while, there may be more than one organism present. This is termed a mixed growth of doubtful significance. Your doctor may have to order another MSU. If there are strong second and third organisms present, the MSU may have been contaminated from extra outside factors and an unclean sample, again necessitating another MSU. **Less than 10,000 organisms per millilitre** may be present in normal urine from people without symptoms, and would be recorded as a technical absence of infection. **However, this may still be an infection, a chronic infection, though not technically counted as such by the lab.**

Do follow my previous instructions for collecting a clean MSU, because you will help the laboratory to give an initially accurate result saving a lot of time and money, frustration and pain.

After plating the urine samples, the smeared plates are stacked on top of each other upside down so that any condensation forming on the inside of the lid does not drop into the growing bacteria to dilute them. At the end of the day all the plates are racked and taken to the Hot Room. Here, at 37˚C / 98.6˚F (body temperature), the organisms have all night to reproduce.

The remaining urine in each sample jar is refrigerated for two more days, in case more is required for a different test. If not, then after two days the jars are autoclaved (whizzed round) until sterile; the urine, now clear of organisms, is thrown down the plug-hole; and the empty jars are sent off to be incinerated.

In the mean time, the microbiologists have decided from the doctors' forms which additional samples should also have microscopy (examination under a microscope.)

The MLSO then collects those sample jars chosen by the microbiologists for microscopy. Wearing protective gloves, he or she shakes up the contents of each jar again, then dips the discardable end of a fixed-volume (60-microlitre) Finn pipette into Rita's urine specimen jar. The pipette sucks up exactly 60 microlitres of her urine, then releases it into a small hole in a flat-bottomed tray.

The MLSO then uses an *inverted* microscope to look at the urine from *underneath* so that the organisms can be clearly seen. The MLSO is looking for pus cells, red cells, squamous cells, casts and crystals.

Pus cells	Indicate inflammation
Red cells	Indicate blood
Squamous cells	Are broken oil skin cells from, say, the urethral or vaginal lining.
Casts from kidney tissues	Indicate disease of the kidneys
Crystals	Occur in certain urological conditions

Whatever the MLSO sees, it is only a visual, the real 'meaty' results of Rita's MSU will be what has grown overnight on the culture plate.

What is seen under the inverted microscope is entered on a very small label to be stuck on the original doctor's form.

Pus cells are counted; if above 10 cells show, it is a probable UTI (urinary tract infection).

If Red and Squamous cells are seen, then 10 cells = Few; under 100 cells = Moderate, over 100 cells = Numerous, indicating the likelihood of infection.

All the doctors' forms, now with a lot of information gathering on them, are put in order of urine specimen number to await the addition of the next day's plate culture growth report.

At about 9 a.m. the next morning, the MLSO begins examining the differential culture plates, writing in brief on the back of the form what has been found. Each plate and its four cultures are made clearly visible under a strong light. The MLSO is trained to spot the obvious bacterial groups and then to implement further instant tests and more overnight tests if the precise organism growth has not yet revealed itself.

In the laboratory, approximately 70 per cent of all positive urine samples show a Coliform growth. Next come *Staphylococcus, Streptococcus, Pseudomomas, Proteus and Klebsiella*, making up between them the other 30 per cent. All are bacteria from our *own* bowels.

A lot of mixed infections come up and, despite the obvious differences to the naked eye of sparse, medium or heavy plate organism growth, the laboratory protocol (procedure) dictates that no further testing is done and the result then given as it stands to the requesting doctor. The understanding is that the doctor will tell the patient to take another sample, as the mixed infection is felt to be indicative of an unclean specimen. The patient should be taught to take a fresh clean early-morning specimen and to get it to the lab quickly. This does not always happen!

Sympathy antibiotics have probably already been prescribed and taken, even before the sample result has come through! This is bad luck but should not alter the enthusiasm with which specimens are taken early on in infections.

In addition to a tremendous range of bacteria-proving tests, the microbiology laboratory also has to recommend to the patient's doctor an antibiotic to which the bacteria are sensitive:

'*sensitive to*' means bacteria cannot grow or thrive

'*resistant to*' means bacteria can still grow and thrive

So another culture plate is set up on night two or three of the urine sample's stay in the laboratory. This next plate is called a Sensitivity plate; there is room for only six small discs on each plastic Lysed Blood Agar Sensitivity plate. With a laboratory loop the MLSO scrapes up a tiny amount of the organisms grown on the differential plates overnight and sets it gently down in the centre of the Sensitivity plate. The edge of the plate is spread with a 'control' fully-sensitive organism. Each disc is impregnated with a different antibiotic and set near the outer edge of the plate. Overnight they will grow around 'friendly' antibiotics but appear to stay away from 'unfriendly' ones. Hence they are either 'resistant to' or 'sensitive to' an antibiotic.

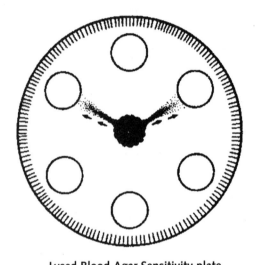

Lysed Blood Agar Sensitivity plate

This also spends a night in the Hot Room at 37°C/98.6°F.

There are four main sets/groups of antibiotics tested on the Sensitivity plate. Each of the four sets contains up to six antibiotics which are especially good for fighting urinary infections. Most organisms are sensitive to all of these. Second-degree and third-degree sets are used for resistant coliforms and pseudomonas; fourth degree sets for staphlyococci.

Set 1	Set 2
Ampicillin/Amoxycillin	Ampicillin/Amoxycillin
Sulphamethoxazole	Augmentin
Trimethoprim	Gentamicin
Nalidixic Acid	Ciproflaoxacin
Nitrofurantoin	Cefuroxime
Caphadroxil	Teicoplanin

Set 3
Azlocillin
Azlocillin
Netilmicin
Amikacin
Ceftazidime

Set 4
Azlocillin
Penicillin
Methicillin (Flucloxacillin)
Novibiocin
Rifampicin
Tetracycline
Fusidic Acid

Other sets of less well-known antibiotics can be tested when required, or the MLSO can arrange for just one special antibiotic to be tested by itself.

It is while these professionals are at work on her sample that Rita should use the first-aid management process to keep herself as comfortable as possible until the results are through. 'Sympathy' broad spectrum antibiotics may be taken at this time.

Once the full range of tests is accomplished, your doctor is sent the report, the laboratory computer updated with the final diagnosis and the old culture plates autoclaved and incinerated.

CHAPTER FOUR

Where Do The Bacteria Come From?

The vast majority of bacteria causing urinary infection come from the victim's own intestines and bowels, 'the intestinal tract' as doctors call it. Others may come from dirty swimming pools, dirty sexual partners, dirty sexual partner's underwear and towels, dirty toilet seats and elsewhere.

How Do Bacteria Get Into the Intestines?

All bacterial micro-organisms found in the gut are also present in the air, on the ground and in all water. They enter the food chain at many points. They could be resting on a plate of food, or introduced by contaminated hands during food preparation, or through liquid intake. When the weather is humid and moist, they breed in greater numbers and we even breathe them in! We obviously also eat them as a matter of daily habit, but we first acquire them at birth or very shortly afterwards from the air, the birth environment and our mother's milk. Micro-organisms enter into our intestines and stay there for the rest of our days! They are known then as 'the normal flora', an essential part of our resistance to infection.

Amounts and kinds of bacteria present in our system change continually. Old bacteria die and new ones reproduce. Keeping balanced in relation to one another is what keeps them all occupied. If one lot overgrows, the others attack - if they don't, the body may succumb to an overwhelming bacterial infection; left untreated by antibiotics this would lead to the death of the person and the death of the other bacterial colonies. So they fight within us for their own survival. We remain totally unaware of all this activity, thank goodness!

Whilst busily occupied with their own life and death, the many groups of enterobacteria (those specifically living in the intestines) cause us no trouble at all. They may even be helpful in breaking down particles of enzymes, proteins, fats and acids which are left at the end of the digestion of food. But trouble does arise if they overgrow, such as if we eat large amounts of carbohydrates (enterobacteria love to eat carbohydrate particles), or if they get outside the intestinal tract where there are fewer colonies of enemy bacteria to fight them off.

Immune-system response is therefore important, so the very young, very old, sick or dying can become terribly ill with enterobacterial overgrowths. Particularly common sites of infections are the lungs and the urinary tract. Lung infections arrive via air, bloodstream or throat; urinary tract infections mostly occur when external perineal bacteria from the bowels travel up and into the urethral tube and bladder. Oral sex can cause oral and sexual bacteria to be swallowed.

Discovery of Bacteria

How on earth has all this unseen life within us been discovered? It cannot be seen with the naked eye, so could the doctors be making it all up?

Until just over a 120 years ago, micro-organisms could not be discovered because the compound microscope had not been invented. Only simple glass lenses with insufficient powers of magnification existed. These simple lenses were first used in the 13th century and no improvements were made to them for another 250 years. Then in the 1650s a Dutchman, Antony Van Leewenhoek, made his own simple lenses to try to satisfy his curiosity about living things like plants, water and scrapings from bad teeth, blood or animal manure.

Lacking a laboratory and without knowledge of culture growth, he couldn't grow organisms, only look at patterns of their colours on seemingly lifeless objects. Those organisms not dying straight away he drew and reported what he could about them, but it was still a pretty hopeless state of affairs. Not until the 19th century with Louis Pasteur, Koch, Weigert, Salomonsen and Hoffman and brilliant additional discoveries from Ehrlich, Loeffler, Ziel and Nielson - were microscopes upgraded and improved. The techniques of growing cultures and of staining slides with colours to show up colourless bacteria then enabled the modern science of microbiology to really take off.

The culture plates described in the previous chapter were first invented by Oscar Brefeld in 1872, who was later helped by Frau Hesse and a Mr. Petri, who came up with the final version in 1882 of what is still used in laboratories today for the growing/cultivating of bacteria. They are even known as Petri plates (or dishes)!

It is only within the last 120 years that scientists have discovered the world of unseen bacteria. For each species and sub-species scientists have invented names and numbers for identifying and referencing them. And discovery is continuous.

Bacteria Colonising Intestines

We know that feces carry solid waste material out of our bodies; we are not going to investigate it all here. What we are interested in are the six main groups of aerobic (oxygen-loving) bacteria that cause infections of the urine, urethra and bladder. These can mount higher up the system into the kidneys and then into the bloodstream so that you may feel dreadfully unwell all over.

A normal, bacterially balanced, easily passed stool doesn't smell nasty, but if you are ill with some kind of infection or virus it may be quite offensive. During the acute phase of mercury poisoning from my amalgams and added gold caps, both stools and urine literally stank. I know now that this was because of methyl mercury being formed during metal corrosion. If stools and urine are always offensive this is abnormal.

The groups of bacteria are members of a 'super-group' called Enterobacteriaceae, which includes:

Escherichia Coliforms
Klebsiella
Proteus
(which are part of the *Coliform* group)
Pseudomonas
Staphylococcus
Streptococcus
(which are part of the *Coccus* group)

but over 100 other types of organisms are quite normally found in stool analyses.

Coliforms

Coliforms sub-divide into many numbered individual kinds. The commonest is *Escherichia coli*, and within that group the O-numbers of 1, 2, 6, 7, 11, 15 and 75 cause more urinary infections than others. Why the name 'Escherichia'? In 1866 a man in Germany called Herr Escherich discovered these rod-shaped bacteria in the feces of babies. Although he called them *Bacillus*, we now know them as coliforms and the commonest variety as Escherichia coli.

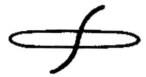

A coliform

Rod-shaped coliforms are, of course, only microscopic in size. They are measured in microns (one micron is a thousandth of a millimetre). Coliforms are measured at about 1 unit wide and 5-8 units long. Swimming in moisture, they multiply extremely quickly, dividing every 20 minutes under best conditions. After 24 hours on the differential plate in the Hot Room at 37°C/98.6°F, the culture plate is covered in coliforms, as easily obvious to the naked eye as the letters on this page.

Most coliforms are very mobile because of their *flagellae*, which act as oars running the width of the rod from side to side. As well as needing a moist or wet environment, food -in the form of sugars of all sorts, carbohydrates and proteins, all of which are present from human ingestion in our intestines- is essential to their survival. Coliforms reproduce themselves continuously by dividing and subdividing, the rate dependent upon the conditions in our intestines, i.e. the meals we have eaten in the past 24 hours, or how well our immune system is functioning to keep the colony numbers self-regulatory. If we are ill already, the coliform colonies will overgrow because other bacteria are too busy with the illness to find time to fight the coliforms off.

Our body temperature of 37°C/98.6°F, in which the microbiologists grow laboratory cultures of coliforms, mimics human conditions. Higher temperatures may produce a higher rate of bacterial reproduction, lower body temperatures may slow down the bacterial activity.

What all this shows is that human beings provide the perfect environment for some bacterial growth. Everything these little bugs want, we can provide in never-ending amounts. One quite interesting point is that once the coliforms are overgrowing, reducing stocks of proteins, etc., they die because of their own overgrowth. Some doctors have shrugged off urinary infections as 'self-regulating' in that after three or four days bacteria are dying or dead having so depleted their own living conditions that reproduction becomes unsustainable.

I seem to remember telling these doctors that if they personally had ever had an attack of cystitis they would not want to wait on without treatment or first aid to see if it went away by itself. There is also the risk of infecting the kidneys and adding to scarring throughout the urinary system.

Proteus

Proteus bacteria are rod shaped. They are 0.5 units wide but only 1-3 units long. They swarm together on some culture plates and need their own additional laboratory test since they can resemble the Pseudomonas group of bacteria. Flagellae enable them to swim well in moisture and they prefer temperatures between 20 to 40°C/68 to 104°F. Once inside the bladder they act viciously, repeatedly causing lesions and bleeding from old scars in the lining. Proteus uses urea in urine to make ammonia, which turns urine alkaline (opposite of acid) and excess ammonia sometimes leads to 'infection stone' formation. Alkalanising urine with bicarbonate, or potassium citrate, as mentioned in the first-aid method on pages 15-16, does not therefore inhibit a Proteus infection.

Proteus bacillus

Klebsiella

Klebsiella are bacillae that live singly, seldom joining up except occasionally as twins. They are static souls protecting themselves from frequent attack by other inhabitants of the intestines with a slimy coat. Although living singly, they still form 'singles' colonies on the culture plates! They look more oval in shape than either rod or circular and vary from 0.5-1.0 units wide and 1-3 units long.

Klebsiella bacillus

Growth occurs at 37°C/98.6°F; killing them off would require boiling them for 20 minutes of 60°C/140°F. I find all these temperatures and times staggering: for me they beg the question of what temperature a human being would finally die at if boiled!

Cocci

Staphylococcus

Staphylococcus, part of the Coccus group, looks quite different from coliforms and measures only 1 unit in diameter, being circular in shape. Staphs, as we will call them, tend to cluster together, much like a diamond-cluster engagement ring. There are three main groups of staphs but others do exist.

single coccus   **cluster of cocci**

Staphylococcus

Staphs are part of the normal flora found on healthy skin, particularly in folds of skin like those on the perineum or penile foreskin. In overgrowth staphs create pus; they are also found in boils, nasal infections and lung infections. Some strains may also lead to infection of the blood vessels in bones and resultant osteomyelitis. Bladder catheters are a source of staph infection. Some types of staph cause Urinary Tract Infection more readily than others.

Staphs are one of the main hospital-induced infections, being present in the nasal cavities and colds of hospital staff and patients where warmth and weakened resistance creates an exceptional environment. They can also grow, unlike coliforms, in a wider variety of temperatures ranging from $12°C/53.6°F$ to $45°C/113°F$, and produce great colonies in only 18 hours!

Staphs eat the usual particles of proteins, carbohydrates and sugars, which reach the outer skin surface via either a cut on the skin or a boil. Moist mucous secretions of the nose, throat, lungs, vagina, vulva and perineum and foreskin are rich in bacterial food and transport. If you have a cut and the staph exudes pus, the pus scab acts as a physical barrier to the further spread of staphs but not within the bladder where urine and lack of air prevent scabbing. Staph is so prevalent now, especially in hospitals, that its own geneticism has begun to produce an enzyme that is resistant to most antibiotics.

Streptococcus

Streptococcus looks the same as Staphylococcus but forms up in chains rather than clusters, which is one of the determining differences assessed under the laboratory microscope.

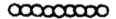

single coccus   **chain of cocci**

Streptococcus

There are three main groups of Streps but, again, many others exist.

Strep Pyogenes and Strep Pneumoniae Both these groups of Streps live in the nasal cavities and throat. If access to the bloodstream has occurred, antibodies will gather at the site and mostly succeed in repelling the invasion. Not always, though, and *Strep pyogenes* infections are responsible for throat and ear infections, local skin infections (anywhere), scarlet fever and childbirth fever. *Strep pneumoniae* will cause upper respiratory infections such as pneumonia, blood sepsis or meningitis.

Strep Fecalis (or *Enterococcus fecalis*, as it is now known) is a really dire one when it comes to urinary infection since, like coliforms, it lives in the bowels on a permanent basis. Once a stool is passed, *Strep fecalis* stays on the perineum, enabling bacterial travel and ultimate penetration of the urethra and bladder, just like coliforms.

Its primary food is sugar but it also draws nutrients from mucous and blood. It, too, can reproduce under low temperatures or high temperatures, making virtually all environments and weather conditions favourable.

Once *streptococci* have invaded the urethra and bladder, growing colonies can cause lesions (cuts or breaks) in the surface skin, encouraging bleeding and the exudation of pus into the urine. With every microscopic or minute lesion, a scar remains to give less resistance to the next bacterial invasion.

Pseudomonas

The strain of *Pseudomonas* bacteria that particularly carries human infections is called *Pseudomonas aeruginosa* and rarely grows in the intestines, skin or throat. It usually erupts into an infection when there is an existing lesion, or when the intestinal balance is poor. Catheters, urethral operations and antibiotics tend to encourage *Pseudomonas*.

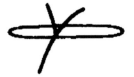

Pseudomonas bacillus

Each rod is thinner than a coliform and shorter in length, measurements being 0.5 units wide and 1.5-3.0 units long. It can also be called Pseudomonas pyocyanea (green pigment) and is a fast mover, having one flagella which branches into three waving 'oars'. It loves the $37°C/98.6°F$ of the laboratory Hot Room but can reproduce at $5°C/41°F$ or anything else up to $45°C/113°F$. A higher temperature will kill it off.

Antibiotics

Perhaps some very generalized information on these medications might round off this chapter nicely.

Antibiotics act in two ways: either by effectively preventing bacteria from reproducing (such action being termed 'bacteriostatic') *or* by actually killing them through bactericidal action.

Of the common antibiotics, Penicillin, Streptomycin and Neomycin act bactericidally. Tetracyclines, Sulphonamides and Chloramphenicol act bacteriostatically.

The action of antibiotics on each strain of bacteria varies enormously. Over the years, scientists working for the major pharmaceutical companies have had to discover and document the precise ways in which bacteria react to each drug and exactly how they are killed off or curtailed.

Patients should be well aware of the general action of broad spectrum treatment because of responding yeast upsurges. Secondary bacterial infections, caused by insufficient or ineffective antibiotics, can rapidly overgrow as a reaction to the death of most of their number and the need to get back to full colony strength.

An obvious additional factor to the laboratory's recommended antibiotic is whether you are allergic to it. Any side effects such as sickness or diarrhoea occurring in the first hours or days of administration should be reported to your doctor and the drug's suitability should be reassessed. You should probably not take any of that class of antibiotic again in the future.

There is also no doubt that these gut bacteria are cunning little bugs! They are quite able, over time, to become resistant by changing genetically or by producing new enzymes able to override drugs. Bacteria learn to adapt faster than pharmaceutical scientists do!

Chlamydia and Candida

Two other organisms are worth a mention here. The first is *Chlamydia*, which we all know about from vaginal swab tests and magazine articles. *Chlamydia trachomatis* is the strain associated with urethritis and cervicitis.

Chlamydia does not inhabit the intestines like the others, but instead acts like a parasite, invading and then setting up home in the cytoplasm of epithelial 'skin' cells.

Chlamydial infection can be transmitted from one person to another.

Transmission is by sexual contact, during which skin cells are passed on and the parasite goes as well. In women, the infection is in the cervix as well as the urethra, so vaginal discharge may be a symptom.

The second extra organism is that well-known fungus called *candida*. Candida/yeast can be present in the bladder and cause cystitis, there is a test available in most large hospitals.

Candida starts out life in exactly the same manner as described for other intestinal inhabitants, but can also be found in all mucous areas of the body. Only when the body becomes debilitated, diabetic or immuno-suppressed from antibiotics, mercury poisoning or other diseases will the candida fungus overgrow. I have written much about candida elsewhere so here I just want to talk about it in terms of the urethra and bladder.

Indwelling urinary catheters may introduce candida to the bladder. Long-term antibiotics and inflammatory lesions of the bladder lining may predispose a woman to bladder Candidosis. Candida is carried in the bloodstream (which has an alkaline pH) and the presence of yeast-infected blood in bladder urine may help maintain the alkalinity, thus providing a welcome habitat.

After antibiotics, bladder urine may carry yeast organisms that have overgrown in the intestine and are being passed out via blood filtration in the kidneys. Candida is often cited on death certificates as a contributory factor in severely sick patients. It is capable of travelling to every organ of the body in blood vessels and needs to be taken more seriously by microbiologists and doctors in relation to the great social and physical suffering which vaginal thrush can cause. Candidal infiltration of gut lining encourages hyphae to branch out and embed in tissue. Scarring and weakening tissue inhibit healthy digestion.

Controlling Bacteria

Artificial control of bacteria is expensive in terms of labour, time, equipment, sampling, doctors, paperwork, antibiotics and patients' suffering. If bacteria are normally in our intestines and *normally* cause no trouble except when outside the intestines and doing some perineal travelling, there must be some way, not involving microbiological and pharmaceutical intervention to prevent that bacterial travel, trouble and expense. Apart from a debilitating course of antibiotics, what other course of action can you, the patient, take?

CHAPTER FIVE

5 How Can I Stop The Bacteria?

Quite simply, you can't 'stop' bacteria, nor should vaccination be used - but you can control them. Such bacteria have been with us since we were primevally formed.

I am going to divide this chapter into two parts. The first is to show research done in the 1960s by the renowned Royal Navy Surgeon Captain Cleave. The second part offers practical hygiene procedures to prevent urinary infections - my own discovery arrived at over years of trial and error.

We Are What We Eat

Surgeon Captain Cleave, now deceased, was a much travelled Royal Navy surgeon with an interest in research as the sometime Director of Medical Research at the Royal Navy Medical School in Hampshire. He spent most of his medical life being fascinated by the health of the naval men under his care and on shore leave abroad he amused himself by collecting data on the dietary habits of many different races of people, most frequently on the Indian and African continents. He would compare these with the diets of his own Western naval patients. After the Second World War he began to witness increasing ill health in the Western world and among his men.

Food Refining

What we eat, which ends up as faeces in our bowels, starts out by entering our mouths. The process of refining the tough fibres from cereals, pulses, fruits and vegetables has very slowly evolved since Anglo-Saxon times, but quickened up from the 19th century when presumably the Industrial Revolution and an easier export/import trade turned foodstuffs into a money-making industry. The continuing addition of refined white sugars to virtually every meal is a much discussed topic by health educators.

As long ago as 500 BC, white flour, sieved and bleached to remove the brown fibrous outer husks, was originally known only to the stomachs of well-to-do Greek farmers and nobility. When sugar refining began from sugar cane and sugar beet it was too laborious to provide for general consumption, so only the rich had access to it. Sugar wasn't exported to Britain until the 12th century, but from the end of the 18th century consumption rates rocketed, reaching all areas of society.

Hippocrates in his medical school on Kos used white flour specifically as a medicine for arresting diarrhoea, since he noticed how much more slowly it passed through a patient's gut into the feces. Refined white flour is much stickier when mixed in moisture and stays longer in the intestines. As the starch in the flour ferments into sugar, that sugar spends longer in the intestines enabling all bacteria normally resident in the intestines to multiply more easily, since they are not constantly kept on the move.

Thus the 'sweet tooth' is a multi-million pound industry the world over - drinks and sweets manufacturers being two of the major monetary beneficiaries.

Apart from the rise in the incidence of tooth decay that accompanies the increased consumption of white flour and white sugar, all sorts of illnesses connected with the digestive process have increased in prevalence, including ulcers, irritable bowel syndrome, diverticulitis, varicose veins, hemorrhoids, obesity, candida, diabetes and urinary infections. Surgeon Captain Cleave produced dozens of charts and diagrams to support all this, and indeed we all know that refined foods are less good for us, even if we don't technically know why. Peristaltic waves are muscular ripples or contractions of the colon walls pushing feces snake-like along and into the bowels for evacuation.

If peristaltic waves are slowed, constipation results and bacterial multiplication increases. Human geneticism cannot cope with bacterial build-up, so the maintenance of a good, healthy digestive system becomes extremely difficult.

Bacterial levels depend largely on how long food processes through intestines and out of the bowels. If it is quick, fewer bacteria thrive but if your system is slow, greater bacterial reproduction results.

Husks on oats and wheat are the fibre which helps maintain a faster, more regular bowel evacuation. But many people are allergic to cereal. Individual experiment is the way to encourage a faster digestion and evacuation. Surgeon Captain Cleave felt that changing from white flour to whole meal flour and the avoidance of all white sugar should be sufficient in itself to get a daily bowel movement, but he recognized that this was dependent upon each person's metabolic rate. There is no doubt that sugar in all forms and from all sources causes constipation. Cut it out and stools become looser and regular. Fresh vegetables and regular fast walking are also very helpful

Regular bowel movements decrease bacterial activity. Most bacteria and toxins work within the intestines to aid digestion but can quickly overgrow and Surgeon Captain Cleave also stresses strongly not to overeat. Bacterial response to large amounts of food is to multiply faster because the food requires larger bacterial colonies to help break it down. In turn, they multiply faster to deal with this extra workload.

Reducing Levels of Coliforms in the Intestines

Three rules exist to help maintain smaller levels of coliforms in the gut:
1. Don't encourage coliform overgrowth by over-eating.
2. Don't eat white flour or sugar as this nourishes coliforms.
3. Don't get constipated as this retains old bacteria.

Eating bran rather than cutting out sugar could cause more constipation. If you only take wheat bran, the ridged colon may clog up with the fine wheat particles which can become impacted and actually create constipation instead of stopping it. Oat bran in porridge is larger and prevents the finer wheat bran from sedimentary build-up. Too many eggs can also be a prime cause of constipation; two or three a week are acceptable. Rice also slows peristalsis and is recommended for diarrhoea. Plenty of **fresh vegetables** provide roughage and minerals and a **good daily walk** agitates the colon.

Massage
Aromatherapists have a digestive massage sequence which promotes peristalsis. It can also be done at home. In bed, lie flat and relax. Using the left hand, rest the palm a little above the left hip bone and using downward movements palpate the colon area with your fingers up and down several times. This 'ripples' the colon and encourages movement of waste products towards the bowels. Have a couple of sessions with the therapist to learn this as well as to enjoy the wonderful delights of the full massage. Colonic Irrigation is not for everyone and is a treatment rather than a daily natural process to help bowel evacuation, it's basically an enema.

Conventional Medicine

Women's urinary infections are still the commonest female problem though self help since 1971 has seen a steep decline in cases approaching the family practitioner. Medical schools are out of touch with the common, simple medical complaints of life and, I believe, often fail their young trainee doctors. High-tech medicine is all the rage, so are more 'unique' illnesses that do not affect so many thousands of patients. Most of us want the illnesses that affect the majority of people to be cured in simple, effective ways. Instead, millions of pounds are poured into new engineering that may help only a handful of people.

Figures from a 1972 survey show the futility of medical procedures:

Q. How many cystoscopies have you had?
A. 774 (between 750 women)
Q. Have you needed further major renal surgery?
A. 50 out of the 750 women needed operations or treatment

So time and money had in effect been wasted on the remaining 724 women. Medical interference is costly and, in the case of urinary infection, unnecessary and ineffective. The quality of your life in this regard lies entirely in your own hands, and those of millions of women around the world like you.

Another survey of doctors in General Practice shows that between 1971 and 1991, a 50% reduction in cystitis from 10% to 5% of all weekly consultations happened during the first twenty years of my campaign for self help and better perineal hygiene.

Personal Hygiene

In many countries, women practise differing methods of hygiene, and many as a result suffer fewer urinary problems than we in the West do. Female hygiene and bladder care is in the hands of the bladder's owner - you!

Over the years of preaching this gospel I have used two methods of washing away the bacteria that cause urinary infections.

The earlier wettened wash-cloth worked for some extra-careful women but was not at all foolproof. Now, Bottle Washing is 100 per cent foolproof for all women, no matter what their social or financial circumstances, if they do it correctly. With qualifications! There are many countries where clean water is absent. Clean water is central to hygiene and good health. We may not like the taste of big city tap water or like its chemical contents, but compared with the water of, say, Calcutta or Lagos it is superb and, what's more:

- There is enough of it
- It is piped into our own homes
- We can make it hot or cold
- It is largely uncontaminated

We do not value water as we should. When you have to wash your whole body in one basinful, twice a week, you quickly learn to value it, I can tell you!

As many of my readers will know, I learned this in Lagos, Nigeria. It was here that I stopped washing my perineum with a wash-cloth. From my first week in Lagos I adopted the brilliant method of bottle washing.

The tap water in our home, like everywhere else in Lagos, was brown and gritty. Within three days I had my first urinary infection in four years despite maintaining my normal rigorous hygiene procedures.

The only thing different was the quality of the tap water. So, watching my stewards each day filtering and boiling this brown liquid and then storing it in old orange drink bottles in the fridge to use for cleaning vegetables, making ice, etc., I found another use for it. Two more bottles were prepared and put beside the toilet in my bathroom. Since that day, in September 1976, I have conquered bacterial cystitis and so have millions of others.

Bottle Washing

Fecal material from your bowels is greasy. Even when you use masses of toilet paper you can never remove microscopic bacterial fecal residue. Think of a frying pan. You can wipe it dry with a whole roll of kitchen paper but it will still smell and be covered with a thin, invisible film of grease.

Invisible fecal residue left on your perineum after a bowel movement is the direct bacterial source giving rise to your urinary infections. As you walk around, the backwards and forwards movements of your legs spreads bacterial residue along the length of the perineum to the vulval area.

Certain extra circumstances help a continued journey of the germs into the urethral opening and up into the bladder.

Those circumstances are:

- poor perineal hygiene
- sexual intercourse
- catheters
- old and thin vulval skin
- physical disabilities or injury
- hemorrhoids
- episiotomy scars
- diarrhoea
- stiff or arthritic limbs

There are lots of other individual lifestyle circumstances which may contribute towards cystitis and still be preventable by Bottle Washing.

Let's take a look at a couple of the circumstances listed above to see exactly how they contribute to urinary infection.

Sexual Intercourse

This is the commonest way for coliform and other fecal bacteria to be helped into the bladder. As intercourse takes place vaginally, the urethra and bladder lying alongside are also pummelled and bruised by the friction. Fecal residue is massaged into the urethral tube and the vaginal entrance. (See Book Two of this Encyclopaedia)

Old and Thin Vulval Skin

All skin ages. From 45 years old it ages faster because female hormone levels decrease. Urethral and vaginal tissues become wrinkly and crinkly as cells that make up a balanced, healthy padding start to break down. Tissue efficiency at throwing off bacterial attacks declines and sexual intercourse may become uncomfortable responding well to Hormone Replacement Therapy either oral or local. If you prefer natural hormone treatments find a Naturopath locally.

Stiff or Arthritic Limbs

In older age, women get stiffer. They cannot bend so easily and some women cannot bathe or wash as well as they used to. They may not even be quite able to use toilet paper properly anymore. Older women need their urine tested reasonably often to spot higher sugar levels, which could denote early signs of diabetes. Coliforms and other fecal bacteria love a diet of sugar, and diabetes provides exactly that. So, in the mildly acidic urine, sugar is an added growth factor. Hormone Replacement Therapy (HRT) can go some way to reverse this process.

How to Wash Effectively

A bath a day for sufferers from urinary infections is no good, for two reasons:

1. You may not be bathing immediately after passing a stool thereby leaving the perineum contaminated indefinitely.
2. If you do bath you will be sitting in a solution of bacteria.
3. Most women 'hope' that simply sitting in bath water is sufficient!

Showering is a little better than bathing, but again is useless unless done straight away, which can be inconvenient.

The timing of when you wash cannot be stressed too firmly. If you bath or shower at 7.45 a.m. but pass a stool **afterwards**, that bacterial residue remains until 7.45 the following morning!

It is far better if you pass a stool at 7.44 a.m. and bath or shower at 7.45; then bacterial residue will lessen.

However, even showering at the right time is not foolproof, because of the way the water drips off the gravity point on the perineum. Standing straight allows shower water to drip off all along the perineum, which means that bacterial residue can run forwards to the vagina. Showering is not a foolproof **perineal** cleaning process. But men must always shower!

Bottle Washing Procedures

Done precisely, bottle washing is 100 per cent effective, quick, costs nothing and can be done anywhere at all, at virtually any time, unless you are in the bushes somewhere!

Full Bottle Washing is for use at home, at work, or out. Vaginal Bottle Washing cleans out sexual liquids after sex and reduces bruising or infection, it also cleans out discharges whilst waiting for swab results.

PROCEDURE 1

Bottle Washing after passing a stool at home
For those with toilet and hand-basin in one room.
You require:
- a basin
- a toilet, well cleaned
- one or two 500-ml (1-pint/20 fl. oz) tonic/soda bottles - not larger or smaller
- a bar of non-perfumed, non-medicated, non-deodorized soap
- a wash-cloth with which to pat yourself dry

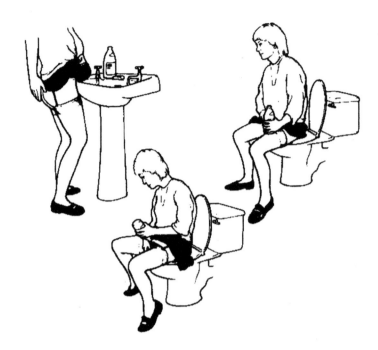

Bottle washing

Now, to Work! Look carefully at the sketches!

1. Pass a stool and use straight, not scrunched up toilet paper (from behind) until this becomes clean.
2. Stand up, flush the toilet but don't pull your pants up.
3. Turn on both hot and cold taps, don't put the basin plug in. Wash your hands and scrub under your nails briefly.
4. Re-soap one hand very well. Still standing up, thoroughly soap the back passage with this very soapy hand. Don't use the bar of soap for this purpose, don't soap further forward, and don't use wipes, cloths or cotton wool.
5. Rinse that hand under the hot, running tap. No plug!
6. Now fill one or two 500-ml soda bottles with very warm water, not lukewarm, but warmer than that. Mix the hot and cold until the temperature in the bottle is right. Turn taps off.
7. Return to the toilet with the bottle(s) and sit down centrally.
8. Position yourself, buttocks apart. Now flop your backbone down (pelvic tilt) and

the anus will follow, being then the lowest part of the perineum in the toilet bowl. Water from the bottle will run downwards into the bowl. It cannot run uphill to the vaginal opening!

9. *From the front,* pour the bottle of very warm water between your legs. Whilst pouring, use your other hand to clean the labia and then reach downwards to help clear away completely all traces of the soap which now contains all the bacteria. Use the second bottle if all the soap hasn't gone. When the soap is off, so are the bacteria.

10. Stand up and pat the perineum dry with the wash-cloth. Keep this apart on its own hook to dry out, even though there aren't any germs on it. They are down the toilet.

Remember, fecal material is greasy. It will only come off with warm water and soap!

COMMON MISTAKES IN BOTTLE WASHING

- Not enough soap to ensure a lather on the anus.
- Using bottles that are too big or too small, or milk bottles that should have been sterilized, or jugs that pour badly. *Only* use 500 ml soda bottles; they have been carefully chosen and researched.
- Not sitting on the toilet with anus as the lowest point.
- Leaning back against the toilet cistern. You just can't reach the back passage from this position and the seat clenches the buttocks, preventing water from a clear backward flow over the soapy anus.
- Using cotton wool or a wash-cloth to put the soap on with. Don't! You contaminate yourself, block up the plumbing, and will miss the skin folds and any hemorrhoids. Only apply soap with your hand so that all nooks and crannies get soapy.
- Using a bidet. *A bidet is dangerous, it spreads bacteria around.*
- Putting the basin plug in and rinsing your hands in a solution of fecal bacteria.
- Not doing it every time you open your bowels and thinking that missing it once will be all right, just you dare!
- Standing in the bath with one leg on the edge and trying to shower the perineum.
- Squatting in the bath - just plain difficult, dangerous and unnecessary.
- Sitting on the edge of the bath instead of the toilet. Pouring the bottle from behind so that fecal germs run forward.

PROCEDURE II

Bottle Washing at work

This is designed for those of you who pass a stool regularly at work, and who have a desk or a locker for personal possessions.

When you buy the 500-ml bottles for use at home, buy two more for work. Also buy a toilet bag that will hold the two bottles, a kitchen paper roll and soap, to leave at work.

1. Take the equipped toilet bag with you to the rest room.
2. First wash your hands very well and then fill the two 500-ml bottles with very warm water.
3. Break off a couple of pieces of kitchen roll, fold in half, pass them once through the hot water tap and soap both of them. Do not use toilet paper; it disintegrates.
4. Go into the stall. Put both bottles down somewhere - perhaps on the floor or a ledge on another piece of kitchen roll. Lodge the two soaped pieces of kitchen roll somewhere clean, e.g. next to the bottles on a piece of kitchen roll.
5. Line the toilet seat with tissue paper, sit down and pass a stool. Use paper as usual.
6. Pick up the soaped kitchen roll pieces and, still sitting, though leaning forward a bit more, soap the back passage well with each piece. Drop them down the toilet behind you.
7. Now 'flop down' so that the back passage is lowest in the pan, this is a pelvic tilt.
8. Pour the bottled warm water down the perineum from the front, using your spare hand to clean away all traces of soap. Use the second bottle if necessary.
9. Break off two more pieces of kitchen roll and dab the perineum dry. If you don't dab you may get minute particles of paper left on the perineum. Kitchen roll is less likely to leave particles but is not as safe as a wash-cloth.
10. Wash hands at the basin and take the toilet bag back to your desk or locker.
11. Remember to remove the tissue paper lining the toilet seat and to leave the stall in a respectable state.

Always refer back to Procedure I if you are in any doubt about the steps involved.

Should you run out of kitchen roll and forget to bring in more, you can use paper towels that are sometimes provided by a wall dispenser - but *don't block the toilet and do NOT use toilet tissue to dry with.* If your cleaning procedure has been less than adequately done, repeat as soon as you are home.

PROCEDURE III

Bottle Washing for those 'caught short'

This is also the method to use if your place of work does not accommodate Procedure II.

The rules bend a great deal here. The one aim is only to do your best. Paper towels may have to do for both the soaping and the rinsing, but such attempts are purely temporary. *Full bottle washing must be done when you arrive home.* Never have sexual intercourse if you have had a bowel movement that day and have not washed afterwards. If you are sexually active it is vital to bottle wash fully in advance of intercourse. Passing wind fecally contaminates the perineum as does normal, constant microscopic anal leakage. We all do this.

Only a downward, backward flow of water successfully removes all soapy residue depositing bacteria in the toilet pan water. Everything else is less effective, probably even wrong.

So, recognizing that fact, I will still run through this procedure point by point for those of you needing emergency washing.

1. Go to the basins first if you are in a strange rest room.
2. Check the paper towel situation. If there are none, abandon the idea of washing until you get home.

or

3. Check your handbag for paper hankies: got some? Four will do.
4. Wash your hands very well.
5. So, with either paper towels or four paper hankies, pass one briefly under the hot tap and then soap it a little. Fold it up again. Alternatively, soap each of two paper hankies, which are less strong.
6. Now wet the remainder, to be used for rinsing.
7. Use the toilet, then paper, then a soapy towel.
8. Still leaning forward, wipe the back passage from behind, pulling a wettened paper towel or paper hankies away and backwards. Fold over and wipe again until all traces of soap have gone. Even so, bits of paper will usually remain. Its not good but better than nothing for a couple of hours.

I personally am quite good at this when I have to be. Just follow logic, get the soap off and remember that you can (and MUST) fully bottle wash back home in an hour or so's time.

Most men fail to use sufficient toilet paper leaving fecal residue all over their underwear! Depending on where they position genitalia within underwear, also whether tight jeans or trousers cause sweating, so this fecal residue can be transferred in intercourse to the tip of the penis and then your vagina!

Check out their underwear and towels (your own also for fecal staining). Men often fail to soap, rinse off or even bother to clean the anal opening in the shower or bath!

Men and women should use lots of soap on the anal opening. *In the shower*, water will follow gravity and run forward into the urethral and vaginal openings so last thing, face the shower and clean off all soapy residue from either vulva (in women) or penis. Two hands are needed to do this so leave the shower up on the wall. *In a bath*, clean and rinse the anus last thing. Stand up to soap it then sit for a moment. Finally, stand again and shower off the whole perineum from front to back.

Other Risky Factors

So you are a young woman with an ordinary bowel movement. I was, once! Now I am older and the mother of two children, with the results of my labours showing clearly upon my perineum! I now own one episiotomy scar and one smallish group of external skin tabs. They are not proper hemorrhoids but the skin no longer sits on the anal orifice as it did in my youthful pre-pregnancy years.

I don't get diarrhoea or loose bowels except if I have a tummy bug, but for many women diarrhoea and irritable bowels can be daily scourges.

Episiotomy Scars

These are miserable. I don't honestly know what's worse: a cut from anus to vagina to shorten a long, strained labour, or a long, strained labour in which pelvic floor muscles lose elasticity and give rise in later years to a prolapsed uterus or a prolapsed bladder.

This episiotomy scar never goes. Every act of intercourse, every bowel strain adds up to further stress and ageing upon it. The long line of scar tissue has less resistance to the movement of bacteria upon it and, as I have said before, it becomes a railway for fast bacterial travel.

It is certainly yet another cause of urinary infection.

Hemorrhoids or Skin Tabs

These are common on the female anal orifice. Young girls can get them if the consistency of stools is very hard; women in pregnancy suffer from them; older women get them from years spent standing up for long periods of time; and really old women get them from sitting down all day.

Depending upon your circumstances, it will pay to have hemorrhoids injected with anti-inflammatory liquid to shrink them. The procedure is uncomfortable but not really painful. You may need some rest and painkillers afterwards, but it improves. Results are usually very good and lasting.

Maybe the hemorrhoids are bad enough to consider surgical removal, or maybe you only need to change your breakfast cereal and stop sugar to encourage looser stools. Suppositories and creams may help temporarily, but if you get to the point of needing these every day, forever, then it might be time to have the hemorrhoids injected.

Irregular and disturbed levels of anal skin provide nooks and crannies in which residual fecal bacteria multiply. Hemorrhoids are a common factor in repeated urinary infections.

Diarrhoea and Irritable Bowels

Well, these things happen in all age groups and for a million reasons. What counts, yet again, in preventing cystitis is whether you wash off that residual fecal bacteria after diarrhoea.

Obviously, if you can sort out the reasons for the upset bowel, you should, but you'll be passing a stool most days anyway. You must wash after every bowel motion all your life. The funeral parlor is going to do me!

Having impressed all these points clearly upon you, what follows are the procedures for bottle washing after sex or for washing out discharge from the vagina.

PROCEDURE IV

Bottle Washing BEFORE sex
This is always a FULL Bottle wash within a half hour of foreplay and intercourse commencing to wash off bacteria.

Bottle Washing AFTER sex
Cleans out sexual liquids that could irritate the vagina and perineum next day, also

reduces inflammation from friction.

Go into the bathroom and:

1. First, wash your hands.
2. Fill up the one or two 500-ml soda bottles with **cool** water this time, which will help to reduce swelling and soreness.
3. Sit on the toilet and pass urine.
4. Re-position yourself until the anus is the lowest part of you in the toilet bowl (pelvic tilt).
5. Pour the cool water from the bottle slowly down the labia and put the longest finger of your spare hand into the vagina. Water will enter with it.
6. When the finger comes out, sexual liquid will, too, in the water.
7. Keep repeating this action until the vagina feels nice and clean again. Five or six times should do the job.
8. Pour a last swill of cool water down the entire perineum and then pat quite dry with your wash-cloth.

The wash-cloth is only for drying, there are no germs on it, and it goes in with other laundry every five days. If you know that your skin is sensitive to washing powders then don't do this. Boil it up in an old saucepan instead. The perineum is also only a small area of skin to dry and doesn't need an unwieldy towel.

Cool water reduces sexual bruising and is a wonderful healer of inflamed skin. You will also have noticed that no soap is used in this procedure. Never use soap frontally; the liquids and moisture of the vagina, vulva and urethra are non-greasy. Only fecal bacteria is greasy enough to need soap. In fact, soap used at the front usually causes many a dose of cystitis from sensitive skin reactions, no matter what soap you use. I must again stress that perineal preparation **before** intercourse is the only way to stop bacterial sexual cystitis. Sex occurs and cystitis starts from the perineal conditions during sex, not when it is all over. Remember, *Perineum Preparatum!*

One more general tip: On no account be tempted to use perfumed, deodorized, coloured or antiseptic soaps on the perineum - elsewhere OK, but not on the perineum.

You might want to make a copy of the Procedure instructions and pin it up in the bathroom until you get it precisely right.

Bottle washing takes only 20 to 30 seconds to do after you have passed a stool, that's all. It is designed not only to be 100 per cent effective in preventing infections but also to be quick. It is quicker than doing your teeth once you do it as I instruct. Don't think that you know better than me, just accept that after years of research and success, I know better than you! I have also been free of trouble for years, by following my own instructions.

Lingering Bacteria

If recurrent attacks seem now to have rolled into one continuous twinge every day of every week, the bottle washing will stop all new incoming fecal bacteria. However, old pockets of inflammation or even bacteria can linger. We must look after the internal side of this as well, so:

1. Drink a glass of water every two hours and also pass urine then. Drink and void keeps urine regularly level and dilute.
2. Take painkillers to calm the upset bladder nerve impulses first thing in the morning and last thing at night.
3. Take potassium citrate or another alkalising agent (as instructed on the packet directions or by your pharmacist) to decrease any acidity. Potter's 'Antitis' (UK brand name) is also helpful.
4. A course of multi-minerals will help the immune system fight and control bacteria.
5. If all is no better after two months, have a three-day course of antibiotics. Keep the self-help going and take further sporadic courses of antibiotics if necessary.
6. I have known severe inflammation to take six months to decrease in some women. Any increase at all in comfort levels should be seen as a good sign.
7. Check out the vagina for any trouble there causing secondary urethral symptoms. Go for a swab.
8. Get checked for Myco-ureaplasma if there is 24 hour pain ongoing, unremitting and for months/years.(See IC Book)
9. LEAVE OFF sweaty clothing, germs love it!

Finally

Everyone leads a different life, has different standards of medical care, differing symptoms and differing resources with which to combat problems. I am always willing to counsel anyone still in difficulties, so don't keep suffering. There is absolutely no reason or excuse for continuing to suffer from cystitis once introduced to my work. After thirty successful years of treating, advising and working on best preventive practices, I know I am quite right. So do most urologists and they are grateful for being able to pass on all this information. So do millions of ex-sufferers; they are now free to live a happy, productive life and become my disciples in this great women's health cause.

I have waged a great war on this misery in many ways, six books, many leaflets, television tours, radio and press items, also a film and a video. You might find my video, for example, very helpful. If you want to contact me for professional reasons or for counselling, please write to the address given at the back of this book.

PART TWO

Non-Bacterial Cystitis

CHAPTER SIX

6 Just Chatting

Medical Obstacles

If, roughly, 80 per cent of all cases of cystitis are caused by bowel germs accessing the bladder, then roughly 20 per cent is caused by something else. This 'something else' can be very simple or it can be a whole parcel of problems that needs unravelling in stages, patiently. It is at this point that the medical profession flaps its hands and finds fashionable phrases such as 'Urethral Syndrome' or 'Interstitial Cystitis'.

Often, medical investigations and patient complicity are very important; often the parcel has been constructed in the first place by medical mishap or ignorance, with the patient bowing to 'the powers that be' in the doctor's surgery or hospital. There are two rules to remember when dealing with medical bureaucracy: first, never agree to surgical intervention unless you have had a second opinion or been for knowledgeable counselling and lengthy discussion, and secondly, keep searching yourself.

There are many other areas of medicine upon which bladder and urinary problems impinge but practitioners nevertheless tend to stick rigidly to the boundaries of their particular speciality. Gynaecologists will seldom discuss or investigate urinary problems and urologists will be reluctant to examine vagina or bowels. Yet it is only too clear that different conditions constantly intermingle within a woman's body.

Those patients coming to me for counselling with this 'parcel' usually have a couple of extra problems preventing a happy outcome, even when they follow my suggestions:

1. The quality of care where they live may already be a difficulty. In addition, local medical knowledge and support may be lacking adding to distress.
2. Lack of funds may prohibit other options outside State services. I recommend all women having private health insurance or taking a bank loan to cover such expenses.

I quite agree that State health services should be perfectly able to help, after all, millions are spent on high-tech operations in terms of both time and resources in order to help a handful of people, so why can't urology and gynaecology take time to pursue more effective treatment of cystitis? Urodynamics, for instance, is a dreadful waste of time, money and correct diagnostic ability in cystitis.

Neither is 'going private' an infallible key to success. It all still depends upon a particular doctor's knowledge and training. Experience with cystitis victims counts a great deal; a 'feel' for the difficulties, a 'hunch' played out and a real understanding of all the interlinking conditions. Everyone involved must be sure of the cause, or causes, and suggestions or treatments only then should be advised.

Taking A Case History

Professional ideas of taking a case history are not the same as my idea of taking one. Mine, of course, also starts with name and address, etc., but then, before any symptoms are taken down, I want to know a lot about a woman's social and work background. Has she a husband/partner? What is his job or hobbies? What does the sufferer do for a living/hobby? I also like to find out about a woman's hours of work, her age, children, details of her home and much more, depending upon her answers as we go along. This question/answer probing provides important diag-nostic details and takes time.

Then I'll ask about her symptoms, when they started, when they come, the day, week or month, any patterns she has noticed, tests she has had done so far, MSU results, operations, and on it goes. Some women can be with me for two and a half hours, some for one if it is a follow-up. Women come from all over Britain, and beyond. Most are desperate, of course, and all go away with a list of ideas and suggestions. It can be a short list or it can run to many points. I don't examine or prescribe, but the difference made when my ideas and suggestions have been put into practice can be quite dramatic. No doctor anywhere has the time or instincts for this approach. It isn't alternative medicine - it is logic, common sense and detective work.

Pioneering

Two historical figures in particular have had similar approaches. The first was Ignaz Philip Semmelweiss, a Hungarian Jewish obstetrician practising in Budapest and Vienna. He began to wonder why, of the two delivery wards in the Rokus hospital, Budapest, his ward had the higher of the heavy maternity death rates. The midwives on the other ward did better. Why? After much research and heartbreak, he came to the idea that it might have something to do with his medical students, who, rather than trained midwives, did the deliveries on his ward. These students would always proceed directly to the delivery ward after carving up dead, putrid bodies in the dissecting room. The lowlier midwives weren't allowed in the dissecting room!

Remember, bacteria were unknown in the mid-18th century. By accident he discovered that when he washed his own hands before assisting at a birth, the mother tended not to die! He introduced a bowl of water and soap at the door of the ward and placed a guard on hand to insist that everyone washed before entering. The death rate began to fall and puerperal fever, which included fecal bacterial infection, began to decline over the next century.

Florence Nightingale wasn't so much a pioneer in fighting one specific illness as leading a fight against the many conditions surrounding illness which tended to exacerbate it and/or its victim's suffering. She was a great believer in hope, reassurance, cleanliness and a preventative approach to illnesses. Environment, both in hospitals and at home, was to her mind very important. She believed in effective sewerage and clean available water. Knowledgeable, kindly nursing was all a part of her ethos.

Both these excellent people had to take a softly, softly approach with their contemporaries. Both had setbacks and scepticism to deal with, yet they were so right and now their work is an integral part of all modern medicine. My own work tries to follow their example. Correct hygiene and common sense are my cornerstones, too. This must be kept up. When you get well, you must tell your doctors and put this book in front of them.

No More Desperation

Only since 1942 have sufferers from cystitis avoided dying. Women everywhere, until the last 50 years or so, became extremely ill and frequently died from urinary problems. Usually it was the rising *E. coli* infections lodging for months at a time in the kidneys, whose working efficiency was impaired as a result. The two World Wars, especially the Second, saw wounds and venereal diseases killing as many off the battleground as on it. Luckily, Alexander Fleming discovered penicillin and so, with the birth of antibiotics, a revolution was brought about in the treatment of infection anywhere in the human body. Kidney disease caused by the rising coliforms was hugely decreased and antibiotic therapy remains the commonest medical response to cystitis.

Antibiotics, as useful as they are, should only be prescribed if infection is proven, but sympathy for the patient, together with her acceptance of 'anything' that will help, usually leads to a course of antibiotics being prescribed anyway. First-aid management of attacks and the many non-bacterial causes of attacks, however, render them (as a sole method of treatment) unacceptable.

Non-Bacterial Cystitis: A Case History

Jane had twingeing by the end of each working day, leading sometimes to attacks of full-blown frequency pain and bleeding when she passed urine. She was a hard pressed personal assistant to a frenetic company chairman. No bacteria was ever found in samples. The trouble began when she started in this job and she was more comfortable at weekends - vital diagnostic clues. Her drinking habits ceased to exist after breakfast except for a cold coffee when she could remember and a glass of wine at lunch if she managed a break. Around 3.00 p.m., time permitting, she had a cup of tea.

No bladder could function with this routine; water is required to dilute the acids and to stop crystals gathering in the urethral tube. Increasing her water intake stopped all her symptoms; antibiotics that had never helped had been proven not necessary and now didn't need to be taken even out of desperation.

This is one of thousands of individual reasons for non-bacterial cystitis. Yet every individual reason can fall into one of the following categories:

- dehydration
- irritation
- chemical contamination
- clothing
- lifestyle in general

Over the next five chapters each of these main groups will be examined, and you will learn how to prevent them from leading to cystitis. Remember: women cause their own cystitis unwittingly. What follows will give you the wits to stop it.

CHAPTER SEVEN

7 Dehydration

Exploitation of Water

The most precious life-sustaining substance on the planet is water. Wars are fought over it and territory mapped out to include access to rivers and seas. It represented the earliest means of long-distance travel, and irrigation canals have been cut into great dry areas allowing more food to be locally grown.

All living plants and creatures need water for cell preservation and blood bulk. Our bodies contain many pints of it as 'capital', if you like; we also require a 'cash flow' of it. It is the cash flow on a daily level that dictates the health of our kidneys, bladder and urethra. We cannot clean *them* as we can the perineum with physical contact; we can only do so by eating and drinking sensibly.

Our diet and liquid intake have evolved from the simplest food and drink sources. Cave people ate berries, greenery, fish and red meats and drank only water and milk until the process of mixing fermented fruits led to the discovery of alcohol. We progressed, learning to work with all sorts of climates and locations to yield popular, staple foods. Life remained fairly simple. Of course, people were often ill from lack of hygiene and gut parasites from eating infected animals, but this became more controllable in the 19th and 20th centuries. Mass food production for town dwellers meant developing ways of preserving food all the way from the farm to the shop shelf and larder.

Food and drink preservation now involves using toxinous insecticides and additives. Even if we could understand the list of contents on food packaging, reading them all is a ridiculously time-consuming effort. So we don't always bother.

Dehydration shows as darker urine, a properly hydrated body passes almost clear urine. Body mass comprises 40-70 per cent water. 75% of muscle and 50% of fat is water and we need anywhere between 2.5 litres a day to 10 litres depending on hot offices, dry air, hot weather, exercise etc. It enters cells and hydrates them if sipped but passes straight through without effect if gulped down.

Tea, coffee, fruit juices, canned drinks and alcoholic beverages contain diuretic caffeine and are false liquids. Liquid can also be taken up from meals, stews, roasts, salads, vegetables, fruits, in tinned foods, frozen or fresh. But sipped water is the best way to keep kidneys, bladder and urethra healthy. The habit of drinking water begins in childhood and should be offered first so that sugared drinks are only treats on Sundays!

- Caffeine in tea, coffee, sweet drinks, etc. is a kidney stimulant.
- Diuretics, especially alcohol and coffee, again encourage a fast output from the kidneys.
- Stress or fear can make adrenaline surge, again stimulating the kidneys.
- Drinking excessively will make the kidneys and bladder speed up and excrete the excess that cannot be used by cells and organs.
- Salt in processed foods and food preparation causes retention of cellular water discouraging regular urinary expulsion and causing a dry bladder and bloating.

Gullibility

All drinks are made attractive to the shopper. Packaging invites shoppers to reach out and buy. Companies need to make money. Nothing wrong in that, but products should be honest and harmless. Children are heavily targeted by marketing departments whose 'Fizzy Pops' leave parents and schools fighting the results: energized, addicted, hyperactive children.

Is Drinking Water Safe?

The UK has seen several outbreaks of Giardia which is common in some European countries. Giardia is a waterborne parasite hard to diagnose, but makes you very unwell, with explosive wind and diarrhoea several times a day. Eradicating the complete infestation can take many weeks, and has to be accompanied by close attention to diet - no red meat and not a drop of coffee or alcohol. Strong antibiotics may work for some but grapefruit seed extract is also helpful.

Tap water in the UK is already loaded with cleansing chemicals and metals often barely above recommended safety levels. A strong resilient gut is needed to overcome possible reactions to these cleansers, yet at the same time no one wants a return to the days when water was so infested that everyone had worms and parasites.

I now use a cartridge water-filter system called the Franke Triflow System from John Lewis stores which contains the lowest traces of silver but still use tap water for dishwashing. One Christmas, my son gave me a Brita water filter jug with a replaceable filter cartridge. Ten days later I became very ill from the silver used to cleanse and filter the water. I became weak, dizzy and had strong stomach pains even after only one mouthful. It was this final clue that led directly to recognising mercury poisoning from fillings because of the heavy silver presence in Brita. Reverse Osmosis systems or distilled water are far better than metalised purifiers.

Capital Savings and Cash Flow

The point at which our bodies reach dehydration can vary. Account must be taken of weather conditions (hot or cold), sweating, fevers, exercise, certain illnesses, alcohol intake, whether we even want to drink. I know women who aren't in the habit of drinking. They just can't be bothered. They are too busy or they forget. Full dehydration, a level rarely reached except during drought or in those with chronic diarrhoea, can lead to death. The kidneys draw upon the contents of other cells and organs to help them continue filtering impurities out of the blood. Finally, when such capital supplies are exhausted, kidney function ceases. The end result of continuous diuretic activity is lowered body liquid levels. The natural inclination then to feel thirsty is the body's effort to balance and replace these lost liquids for its own good.

Failure to drink sufficient amounts of water creates a continuously lower level at which the kidneys cannot work. Without enough, they cannot dilute urine which carries impurities, such as acids and enzymes which have completed their tasks in the kidneys. These can be very strong if undiluted.

Bladder Function and Reaction

Rejected substances all flow in urine down a tube from each kidney called a ureter. Gravity propels droplets every few seconds towards a valve which will only open when a certain amount of urine has gathered behind it. This liquid weight then stimulates the valve to open allowing urine down into the bladder The bladder is a storage facility. It has no other function. Why then can it be such a painful and problem-prone organ?

It is painful because without exceptional sensitivity it wouldn't know when it was full. An exploding bladder isn't a good idea! So nerve endings in the bladder are virtually surface-based and super-responsive. What we put into our digestive system and what we allow up into the bladder via the urethra from outside are major influences governing many bladder problems.

Receiving the results of a night's bar drinking, the bladder must expel liquid as often as it fills up. Bacterial invasion prompts ejection response, too. If you get a fever from a virus or infection, the bladder's reaction to excrete and expel the toxins is part of the body's defence mechanism. In addition to these come all manner of situations that set up reactions.

Insufficient liquid intake decreases bladder urinary output but crystallization of the bladder lining and urethral lining by deposits of uric acid can cause pain. Crystal formation, comprising uric acid, many filtered toxins and waste products, settles and adheres to these sensitive surfaces.

Once settling, the contents of acidic crystals, now in contact with super-sensitive nerve endings, will activate defence mechanisms. Mild twingeing, spasms and shudders may signal a need for the bathroom. So then you pass a small, dark quantity, which may or may not hurt, like a cystitis attack, and could leave you feeling as though you need to go again soon after. Frequency and inflammation lead to an increase in discomfort, sufficient to make you think you have proper cystitis.

Sensible Drinking

Think back over the past few days. Have you drunk the suggested 3-4 pints (60-80 fl. oz/1.5-2 litres) of the day's kidney liquid cash flow at regular intervals? Perhaps you have, but perhaps your body has required even more liquid than normal of late. Have you been working out, have you gone dancing, do you have a cold, have you been rushing around at work, have you had lengthy sex, eaten a Chinese meal with lots of monosodium glutamate a salty additive used in many Chinese dishes, taken a plane trip, got cold at the bus stop, drunk too much coffee? The list is endless because all of us lead different lives, but such factors can, for many women, make the difference between twingeing and comfort.

Listen to what your body dictates. Drink more if you feel thirsty. Drink regularly anyway. Don't let crystals and acidity compromise your urinary system. Dehydration in all its forms is hazardous, and failure to empty the bladder at reasonable intervals is careless. Value your bladder by drinking and voiding regularly.

'Not Quite Right'

If you have found the basic reason(s) for your attacks of cystitis but you can still tell that things are 'not quite right', inflamed skin, either in the bladder or urethra, may still be sore. Internal healing can take a while. Some women recover quickly, others slowly; some so slowly that recovery is unnoticeable for the first weeks. Sometimes it can be helpful to have kept a 'journal' of symptoms, etc. This can help in counselling when a return visit occurs when listing changes can be uplifting and encouraging.

Sometimes adjustments, fine tuning, in the already improving circumstances can make quite a leap in further symptom reduction.

Joanna had come for counselling on her attacks of cystitis, which had regularly ruined her new sexual relationship. We had sorted it all out and she'd had her first sexual holiday in three years! Her slight remaining problem was that passing urine afterwards often didn't 'produce' urine. In order to reduce sexual bruising, I always recommend that the bowels be opened daily and that a full bladder be emptied before sex. This she was happy to comply with, but often sex was short about half-an-hour, and afterwards, when she went to the toilet, there wasn't enough urine ready to be voided. Since most of the sex was occurring at night, the 8 to 10 hours or so of sleep that followed until 7.30 or 8.00 next morning made that next, early morning excretion a bit sorer than she was happy with.

I helped her to 'fine-tune' it by advising a small drink just before sex. This would enable more post-sex urinary excretion, as indeed it did. No matter how little is passed, it must be passed to de-traumatize the 'shocked' bladder and get it settled. A small glass of water after sex does help the early morning urine excretion to be paler or more comfortable. Sex uses up a lot of energy. Sweating, orgasms and natural vaginal lubrication all help remove cell liquid and excite the kidneys. Replace the lost liquids and restore urinary balance, or cystitis, effectively from dehydration, may start.

Checklist for Dehydration

If you think that the cause of your sort of cystitis could be due to poor liquid intake, check;

1. Have you drunk three pints today, at reasonably regular intervals? One or two heavy liquid sessions are not regular, gentle inputs. Such sessions in themselves overwork the kidneys and excess is simply sent straight to the bladder. Some liquid needs to be allocated for cell and organ storage, as well as for urine bulk.

Downing liquid in a heavy 'cash flow' session won't allow for this as efficiently as regular small amounts.

2. Are your urine samples always negative? Of course, there are mountainous reasons for negative results as well as dehydration, but you still need to know that the cystitis is definitely non-bacterial.

3. Do twinges seem to start towards midday or late afternoon? Maybe they are constant? This can mean intake is too low during the morning or afternoon. Often sensations decrease once a woman is at home and drinking sensibly. Teachers can be very prone to this, as can store staff working under hot lights. Days off or holidays never seem to give trouble and are therefore great clues.

4. Is the first morning sample dark and stinging? Look closely at your previous evening's liquid intake and social activities. Perhaps you drank a lot and got up a few times in the night? By 7.30 a.m. there may be nothing left to pass. You must replace and rework the bladder function straight away, or a drying urethra may signal its unhappiness. Perhaps you didn't drink quite enough during the evening.

5. When you are off shift/duty/work, do you get twinges? Do they occur only at work? Do you drink regularly and void at work? If not, look to convenient points when you may increase drinking.

6. Coffee at work is all too common. Stop it for a week and see whether the twinges stop. If this works, allow yourself one weak coffee a day. Otherwise, a bottle of water in your desk will be a great help. No amount of workload or dutiful behaviour should cause ill-health. It is just not worth it.

If you do start a real attack of cystitis and you are pretty sure it is because of dehydration due to lack of liquid, you are best advised to follow the three-hour management programme. Do everything as recommended, including the MSU sample (better safe than sorry!).

Cystitis caused by dehydration will respond very quickly to the management programme and clear up completely in the three hours. It may teach you a valuable lesson about not becoming careless. Women prone to cystitis occasionally need a lesson if they have let themselves down, and nothing pulls them up faster than another attack. It is a reminder from their kidneys, bladder and urethra that careful management, not risk-taking is best.

Antibiotics cannot help cystitis caused by dehydration, nor will they do anything to counteract dehydration. Antibiotics only work against an attack of cystitis caused by germs, nothing else. Don't rely on pills unless there is a background medical condition, such as the lack of estrogen that comes with the menopause/a hysterectomy or old age. Cystitis is mainly self-imposed and preventable by the patient. This understanding is the greatest advance since antibiotics stopped us from dying of it. Antibiotics don't stop attacks from starting nor do they work against non-bacterial causes; it is patient's awareness, prevention and lifestyle making dramatic improvements over previous medical failures. It is up to you!

CHAPTER EIGHT

8 Irritation

Don't Scratch!

If there's an irritation somewhere on your skin, it is natural to want to scratch it but if you scratch until you bleed, blood vessels will spread the cause of irritation to other sites. All of us have done this at some time or other. My own worst times were during my cystitis years, 1966-1971 when continuous antibiotics, heat from baths, bedding, underwear, trousers and my husband lying next to me were agonizing. In those years I woke us both during the night, scratching until blood ran quite freely. Scratching was unstoppable and getting up to dab with cold water in the bathroom was the only thing I could do to wrench myself out of it. It still didn't help much.

Constant scratching damaged a patch of labial skin where fungus rooted for years needing constant attention and calming creams. It did go finally. Irritation anywhere along the perineum and inside the vagina, urethra, bladder or bowels brings additional difficulties. The most obvious ones are:

- It is too embarrassing to try to alleviate in front of anyone.
- No one can see it except yourself in the privacy of the bathroom.
- Much of it is internal, invisible and insufferable.
- Even walking round the house is uncomfortable.

There's another really important rule here for all women: *Don't put any old cream, ointment or antiseptic on the vulval area!*

Forget the adverts for 'intimate' creams; they are very deceptive and mostly worsen the situation either immediately or a few hours later. Only three things make any difference at all:

1. Finding the cause of the irritation as quickly as you can.
2. Resting - no walking.

3. Using a cool water bottle wash or even giving it a few minutes of the 'frozen pea bag' treatment. (Small size bag of frozen peas, wrapped in a clean cloth; don't ever eat the peas).

Causes

Until you are really aware of the specific cause for the particular irritation bothering you, any cream or pill is a matter of experiment and likely failure. Don't think the doctor is a fountain of knowledge guaranteeing diagnosis and treatment, he is no better qualified than you, since only you feel the irritation. You must clearly explain and clearly show the symptoms.

On the couch, point to it if possible; tell when it started and whether you have experienced it before.

Bowel Irritation

Bowel irritation is usually caused by foods or drinks. Irritation in the intestines, which lead into the bowel, can be due to either diarrhoea or constipation. Intestines can react within a couple of hours to something they don't like. It is very individual, this allergy/sensitivity business. Most of us understand that cabbage, broccoli, peas and beans cause wind and bloating; not all of us double up with stomach pain when eating certain sorts of ice-cream or drinking coffee! Mercury leaching from fillings is also a known intestinal aggravant.

The main allergy *groups of foods* are:

- Cereals - wheat, barley, oats, corn
- Pips and nuts — tomatoes, peanuts, pecans, grapes, etc.
- Dairy products - milk, butter, yoghurt, cream, cheese, etc.
- Pulses - lentils, peas, beans
- Moulds - yeasts, fungi, cheeses
- Spices, chemical additives like Aspartame and Tartrazine, E types, hormones, many others
- Fruits - citrus mostly - oranges, limes, grapefruits, lemons, citric acids, etc.
- Shellfish - lobster, crab, prawns, oysters, mussels, etc.
- Mercury is common to all fish and fish products
- Many additives, heavy metals, environmental toxins

Any or many can upset individual people.

Bowels excrete solid body wastes bound up by mucous and liquids which, unless bottle-washed off afterwards, remain to cause irritation. Any substances to which you are sensitive can get into the vagina and bladder via fecal residue. But the main entry and reactions occur as the intestines sieve and sort valuable substances from other toxic or allergenic food particles. Liquids are also sorted either for excretion or for storage in cell tissues.

Bladder Irritation

Bladder super-sensitivity can be very great in some women. Whether it is a diuretic substance like alcohol or mercury, or an infection/virus arriving via the bloodstream, the bladder receives it and decides whether it is friend or foe.

Suppose you have such an irritating substance or liquid in your daily diet. It might have newly arrived because of a new change in your lifestyle. Perhaps you are a young mum and do the mercury tuna sandwich /cake flour routine now for children's teatime! Perhaps the new boyfriend smothers the candlelight dinners with black pepper or Chilli! Perhaps in winter you are heavily into hot chocolate with cream! The list is endless for all ages and all situations. Just try to find what is different now from when you were well without a sensitive, excitable bladder.

Finding the cause/s of your bladder trouble is a little easier if symptoms are infrequent. Then look back anywhere within the past 24 hours and see if you have eaten or drunk something slightly different. Maybe there is a favourite fish 'n' chip shop on the way home from your weekly Thursday hairdressing or business trip. Is it the same fish you choose each time, or could it be that the frying oil is nut-based (rather than vegetable-based) and nuts upset you? So Thursday night you make more trips to the bathroom and by Friday morning, the bladder nerve endings are well and truly signalling trouble. Fish is also the highest food source of mercury followed by mushrooms and you may react to both.

Only an allergy specialist can begin sorting you out. Have a go yourself first by observing your eating and drinking habits carefully.

When you think you might have an idea of the culprit, experiment with the food or drink and monitor your response. If the problem is continuous, look at the foods and drinks you eat on a regular basis, such as, for example, breakfast cereals, milk, fruit, chocolate, toast, cheese, mushrooms, jams, teas. Watch for any patterns, particularly if symptoms decrease at times or stop totally for a while. If you have to get up at night, what time was the last drink and what was it? I am still amazed at how many people have a coffee, chocolate or a similar hot drink at 10 p.m.! Obviously they're going to have to get up!

Vaginal Irritation

Not a lot of people, doctors included, know that allergic reactions can influence the vagina. Secondary bladder trouble caused by vaginal problems is discussed later more fully in Chapter 11, but is also worth a mention here.

Mucosal areas all over the body will secrete extra mucous if an allergic substance has entered your body. Noses run, eyes run, and vaginas can become more moist and itchy. Secretions, perhaps from too much fibre (particularly wheat bran) or from being pregnant, can and cause vaginal mucous levels to increase and leak onto clothing. Leakage affects the urethra. Vaginal swabs show negative, the doctor doesn't know what else to do and the frustration is just too much on top of the symptoms. Simply too much fibre can cause all this extra leaking as glandular activity and cell discarding increase. What to do?

If it is fibre:

1. Why is so much fibre being taken?

   a) Because it is just a habit?
   b) Because bowels don't work unless it is taken?

2. Why are the bowels being stubborn?

   c) Because sugar intake is too much for your system?
   d) Because white flour and refined foods are clogging up the intestines?
   e) Because you take insufficient exercise?
   f) Because the wheat bran itself has clogged up the intestines?
   g) Because you overeat or because of mercury influence from teeth fillings?
   h) Because of antibiotics or other medications?

Take any appropriate action on the above, then manage the drip:

- Remove the vaginal discharge and clean out the vagina morning and night as described.

Only after a Full Bottle Wash may you then:

- Fill another 500-ml bottle with lukewarm water.
- Add to this a 1/4-**capful** of Betadine solution, available at any pharmacy. Betadine is a great vaginal comforter.

- Pour this mixture very slowly down the perineum from the front (pelvic tilt position) as for a Vaginal Bottle Wash.
- As the solution is running slowly down, insert the third/longest finger of your other hand up to the cervix and 'hook out' discharge from all round.
- Water and Betadine go inside as well, cleaning and clearing the vaginal walls of sticky, irritative mucous.
- Repeat five or six times until your finger exits clean of any trace of mucous.
- Dry carefully with a wash-cloth not towel or paper.
- Never clean out BEFORE a swab or it will be negative!

By cleaning out the vagina in the morning, dripping won't happen until early evening. Dripping only happens when the vagina can no longer hold the amount of discharge building up within it. If the discharge is no longer dripping out of the vagina and onto your underwear, perineal and urethral soreness decreases. Twingeing inside the urethra will calm down, especially if you increase your liquid intake for an hour or two to clean and calm the nerve responses. Pharmacies may want to sell you the Betadine kit with douche and gloves, but persist, if possible, on first buying the bottle of Betadine alone. It is an iodine-based liquid, but much distilled and diluted. Sore vaginas may not like it to begin with and it is often better to start cautiously with only a 1/4-capful in the 500 ml of water. Increase to half a capful when you like and then a capful if required.

Adverse vaginal secretions setting up irritation at the urethral opening will certainly influence the urethral lining as well. Vaginal swabs are every bit as vital as urine samples for discovering the cause of cystitis and both investigations should be done simultaneously. They seldom are.

I hope that you are beginning to understand how much the bowels and vagina influence the bladder. Keep these in good order and your bladder and urethra will be far healthier.

Yeast in the Bladder

Rather than repeat so many other publications on Yeast/Thrush/Candidiasis/Monilia, I intend here merely to state the rules and give practical tips on avoidance and management.

Thrush breeds in alkalinity, moisture and warmth. Whether this is all provided internally or whether external factors such as a hot bath or sweaty bedding contribute, it matters not. Thrush eats sugar and yeasts, which certainly come primarily from food absorption, but it is also influenced by hormones, glands, enzymes, mercury teeth fillings and other bodily processes.

Yeast is always present in the gut, but upsurges when bacteroides (which break up foods) overgrow Bifidus bacteria (those tending to clean the intestinal lining). There is a constant battle between them and, so long as things are equal, there's no room for candida/thrush to get a hold. Once bacteroides gain ground, however, candida surges.

Understand that thrush of the bladder is a very real condition! It is much overlooked as a cause of cystitis and, sadly, most doctors don't accept it anyway. There is a urine test for it. Urine must be as highly concentrated as possible, preferably a sample taken when you first wake up and microscopy done very quickly. These conditions pose difficulties for State clinics/laboratories but pay, if necessary, and plan sample taking carefully.

Symptoms of bladder thrush may be twingeing and discomfort with urine samples showing no bacteria. The condition will worsen if you eat sugary foods or get hot and you may already have proven vaginal thrush. The appropriate medical treatment is Sporanox (an anti-fungal), for perhaps 10 days to two weeks if severe thrush or lengthy symptoms can be proved. Otherwise Sporanox is a seven-day oral course. Alternatively, a course of Diflucan is also helpful.

Yeast in the Gut and Bowels

Yeast begins in the gut. It is a fungus whose flagellae ('tails') hook onto the lining of the intestines and other sites to obtain nutrients for its reproduction and colonization. Eat sugar, chocolate, cream, yeast, fresh chunks of bread, mushrooms, alcohol, lots of fresh fruit, ice-creams, 'windy' foods, vinegars (French dressings, etc.), fruit juices, canned/bottled drinks or excessive carbohydrates such as flour, rice and pasta, and thrush will surge.

Symptoms for men and women may be bloating, wind, discomfort, gurgling, bleeding bowels. Hemorrhoids may swell and the anus may itch. Elsewhere on the body, the symptoms of a white tongue, sore throat, tiredness, lethargy, dark eyes exuding a whitish discharge, slightly blurred vision, a heavy head, ear exudation, vague tinnitus, dry mouth, tiny white spots on the gums and nasal blockage can all arise from a big gut upsurge.

This gut upsurge causes a general feeling of malaise, contributed to in great part by many lifestyle conditions, such as:

- getting hot through exercise, hot weather, central heating
- being stressed, run-down, tired, slightly or seriously ill, working too hard

- soaking in the bath
- having sex when you or your partner are infected
- wearing tight clothing or nylon/polyester (anything that is not 100 per cent cotton) underwear
- drinking alcohol
- eating the wrong foods
- taking steroids for asthma or other illnesses
- taking antibiotics for any sort of illness; as the effect of antibiotics wanes only after three weeks
- taking anti-depressants long term
- having unbalanced hormone levels for whatever reason
- swimming in chlorinated pools
- having a viral illness such as ME (Myalgic Encephalomylitis) or HIV/AIDS
- being diabetic
- having a mouthful of mercury teeth fillings/gold caps which deplete immune system resources

Individual causes abound, one-offs that come to light only in counselling. Often there will be a cluster of small factors adding to a whole that culminates in upsurge.

Frequently the calendar can be responsible:

- Christmas/birthdays - alcohol
- Easter - finishing off all the chocolate eggs
- Summertime - lots of fresh strawberries/plums/peaches, swimming, jam-making (and tasting)
- Wintertime - layers of extra clothing causing sweating

Pills alone will not work. Reducing and removing the cause will. Responsibility is shared again between patient, practitioner and pharmacy. Ignore this fact and the consequences will be continual trouble and frustration. Nystatin (sold as Mycostatin in the US and Australia) and Diflucan are all right as well, but Sporanox treats systemically - that is, it acts on candida present anywhere in the body, e.g. the sinuses, mouth, gut.

Yeast in the Vagina and Perineum

The vagina and perineum are secondary sites following the main gut source but some women get it before a period.

Symptoms are:
- an itchy, creamy, stringy discharge; or even acute dryness.
- red and swollen labia.
- itchy, swollen, reddened anus.
- acute phases can result in a heavy, purplish swelling of the labia with minimal or no discharge.
- walking can be painful and uncomfortable.
- hemorrhoids may swell and bleed.

What to Do?
1. Get proof of the condition by having a swab taken at the nearest genito-urinary clinic.
2. Eradicate all self-caused factors. I mean it! All of them!
3. Go to bed or take to your sofa in a long skirt, with no underwear, for as long as it takes.
4. Cut pubic hair to 1 in (2 1/2 cm)
5. Cool-water bottle-wash the vagina three times a day. If vinegar in the bottle helps you, then add a capful to acidize vaginal mucous.
6. Before a period insert an acid vaginal jelly to maintain acidity and reduce alkalinity.
7. Take only three soup-spoonsful of a Bifidus-added plain live yoghurt 20 minutes **before** meals.
8. Go gently with acidophilus capsules, they are strong.
9. Increase liquid intake to prevent thrush rising into the urethra.
10. Don't walk, exercise in the gym or have sex.
11. Take oral anti-fungal medication (e.g. Sporanox) and a course of pessaries.
12. Insert the pessary at night, once you are in bed - and don't move afterwards!
13. The pessary must be pressed up against the cervix, not lower. Wear a sanitary towel.
14. Do you still need the steroids or antibiotics? Assessment is important.
15. Have mercury fillings SAFELY removed with a specific method used by mercury-free dentists.

Menopausal/Advanced Age/Hysterectomy Irritation

Women coming to me who fall into one or more of these categories usually use the words 'deep irritation', 'dull pain', 'constant twingeing', 'dragging' or 'soreness' to describe their symptoms. They pinpoint external and/or internal sources of their discomfort.

Additionally, they may complain of aching wrists, neck and knees; tiredness, disturbed sleep; attacks of either bacterial or non-bacterial cystitis that only commenced with the menopause/after their hysterectomy; hot flushes; loss of libido; sweats and, of course, irregular periods (if they are still having them at all).

Hormone Replacement Therapy (HRT), if appropriate, can alleviate or lessen all these symptoms, not just the irritation and cystitis. If the first HRT prescribed isn't quite right, there are many more. Here are other ways of taking HRT:

- vaginal hormone creams
- oral tablets
- patches
- implants
- injections

Of course HRT is not the answer for all women, nor is it always needed but it is increasingly used to prevent osteoporosis and Strokes. Heavy mercury presence from 'saved' and numerous fillings at this age can influence hormones and deplete calcium and magnesium from bones.

Bacterial Cystitis in Older Women

This is common to one-third of older women because a variety of factors, including:

- Stiff, arthritic joints preventing personal perineal washing
- ageing, atrophied perineal skin encouraging bacterial settlement
- diabetes or raised sugar levels causing thrush and urinary soreness
- Urinary catheters
- dirty commodes in homes and hospitals

The answers lie in HRT, mineral and vitamin intake, sugar control, regular walks, careful perineal hygiene using bottle washing not wash-cloths or sponges which retain bacteria.

Environment

Our environment these days is much influenced by fads and fashions. Consumer gullibility is again the key. Bubble baths, for example, were not invented for health - they were invented for wealth - and not yours! They irritate any female vulva of any age. Likewise soap - it has got to be white, unperfumed and unmedicated for use on the anus. Never, ever, soap the vulva (front part). Jeans literally bruise the urethral opening where the seams join. Loose clothing prevents bruising, lets air circulate and protects the body from potentially harmful chemicals.

Irritation in Babies, Little Girls and Teenagers

Bacterial Irritation
Bacterial attacks in youngsters are again caused entirely by an absence of hygiene or by ineffective hygiene procedures. Bottle Washing is inappropriate for small children, but one bath a day should be quite adequate. If it can be done after she has passed a stool, fine. If not, then the daily bath will be important. Soap her back passage thoroughly as she stands up for you, then sit her down and make sure all the soap goes and isn't trapped. Don't soap her vulva - it will sting and it isn't necessary anyway.

Non-bacterial Irritation
Children don't know anything about hygiene. What parents impose upon them is for better or worse. All the little routines, foods, drinks, soaps and timings are fraught with possible trouble-spots leading to sore bottoms. Irritation and soreness followed by pain when they urinate is heartbreaking to watch. The cause lies somewhere in the child's daily life, either at home, at playgroup or at school. Neglecting to investigate and remove this will condemn the child to great unhappiness, lasting drugs, frightening hospital treatments, disrupted sex later on and maybe kidney infection and permanent scarring.

Even without bacteria, rising inflammation still causes the same distress, especially when scarring begins in earnest. Urethra, bladder and kidneys all bear scarring permanently whether it is caused by severe inflammation, infections or surgery. Parental awareness and the playgroup/school situation need sorting out before the child can be sorted out.

Foods and Drinks
Everything I have written about adult food and drink reactions applies to children.

Allergies are often inherited and the new discovery of a gene that can predispose a person to asthma or allergies may illumine these problems as research continues. For now it is a matter of accepting that, either in the same form or slightly different ones, a child can also show signs of allergic reactions.

Check List
- No fruit juices only water or milk. No Aspartame sweetener.
- No sugar-laden canned, cartonned or bottled drinks except as a treat once weekly.
- No sugar-laden foods.
- Limit fruit intake to one piece a day.
- Make sure urine is regularly passed at home and school.
- Change underwear each day.
- No bubble baths or antiseptics in the bath.
- Use only a plain white soap for anal cleaning, none on the vulva.
- No antiseptics or creams on genital skin.
- Beware soreness after swimming in strongly chlorinated pools.
- Make sure she wears cotton knickers and skirts, dresses or loose trousers - never jeans.
- Teach her to clean herself properly after a bowel movement - wiping with toilet paper from behind and not touching the front.
- Check out the washing powder/liquid used in laundering; biological brands in particular can cause irritation.
- Limit flour, breads, pasta, cakes etc.

These are the main guidelines, highlighting the commonest causes of childhood genital irritation and soreness. Take note! When your daughter falls in love and wants sex, it may be down to you if she can't because of urethral damage. Strong words - I make no apologies!

A Couple of Other Triggers

Cold
Windy bus stops, gardening in a stiff breeze, sitting on a stone wall, all seem to affect some women, particularly older ones. It is not bacterial, it is irritation caused by dehydration. The cold stimulus upon kidneys and bladder sets the 'excitor' process off. Urine is passed several times successively more concentrated and acidic. Replacing this excreted liquid with a couple of warm drinks straight away -

maybe even a bath or certainly a warm-up somewhere cosy - should redress the balance and comfort the bladder's 'excited', irritated nerve endings so that soreness and twingeing decrease.

Car Travel

This can be a source of trouble, especially in older, less well sprung cars on long journeys over bad roads. Again, many older women used to cite this as causing bladder irritation. I suspect they had a chronic undiagnosed bladder problem. In any case, with the advent of better cars and better roads I believe this sort of irritation to be on the wane. If it is a bother, then take along a good pillow to sit on, change your car, travel by train, and/or try painkillers to ease the bladder's nerve endings a little.

CHAPTER NINE

9 Chemical Contamination

Practically anything coming in contact with genital skin is man-made. I can hardly name a product that has not been dyed, coloured, treated or added to in some way. Obviously, Rule 1 is: go for the simplest, least colourful, least added-to products you can find.

The Usual Suspects

SOAPS

Only use white, unperfumed, unmedicated, undeodorized soaps. Shower gels, salts, bubble baths, medicated wipes, antiseptic soaps, deodorized soaps and more are packed with chemicals all cited as trouble-makers of genital soreness by sensitive women. Again, always go for the simplest sort and remember never to soap the urethral and vaginal openings. These areas of the body are not greasy and will not have a great colony of bacteria like the anal opening, which certainly has to be cleaned with a soapy hand, as described in the Full Bottle Washing procedure in 'How Can I Stop the Bacteria?'

DEODORANTS

Never deodorize the vulva or anus; wash them properly with bottle washing. Do not use deodorized tampons; do not use panti-liners. Most manufacturers use 'Parfum', check the labels of anything that touches your skin.

How to Reduce Vaginal Odor

- Bottle Wash daily as described.
- Then do a vaginal bottle wash; add the Betadine, occasionally, if necessary.
- Keep pubic hair cut to 1 in / 2.5 cm in length to avoid the retention of odors and fungi.
- Wear cotton underwear.
- Keep the perineum comfortably cool.

- Mercury from teeth fillings also creates odor.
- Check dental health including root canal work.

ANTISEPTICS

Most antiseptics sting and irritate. Never use them on the perineum. Proper bottle washing removes any need for them. Do not use antiseptic for bathroom cleaning, especially never on the toilet seat. Always remove all trace of cleaning fluids with a carefully rinsed cloth, and prevent any splashing up from the pan water when you pass a stool by placing one sheet of toilet paper on the water's surface beforehand. Betadine in Vaginal Bottle Washing is iodine-based and a medication for specific circumstances. Hexacloraphene scrub solutions in hospitals help limit bacteria there, but forbid its use on your perineum especially in labour, just Bottle Wash normally.

SHAMPOOS AND SHOWER GELS

Would you have spotted these as the possible cause of irritation? Either sex using them can risk chemical contamination of the penis or vagina. This might then be transmitted as an irritant during intercourse. Foreskins are often improperly rinsed leaving chemical contamination in the folds. Contamination builds up and transmits regularly into an increasingly sore vagina.

Hair should only be washed over the bath as chemicals inevitably build up in vulval and penile tissues in all age groups. Soreness might start immediately with a new bottle or might build up over several weeks of bath times using a variety of shampoos.

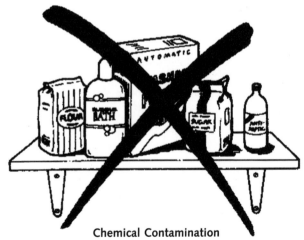

Chemical Contamination

BUBBLE BATHS

Ghastly! A major cause of non-bacterial irritation, soreness, discharge, urethral stinging and cystitis. Use them, buy them at your peril. They should carry a government health warning. I mean it!

WASHING POWDERS/LIQUIDS AND FABRIC SOFTENERS

All or any of them build up in underwear. If you suddenly get a cystitis attack out of the blue, any change of your usual brand of washing powder/liquid or softener is always a good thing to check. Cotton underwear can be boiled clear in successive pans of water to remove contamination.

Looking at Redness

Always have a good look at the perineum when it is 'upset'. Wash your hands and perineum, then lie down and shove a cushion under the buttocks so that this tilts the perineum forwards a bit. Try other positions until, with a mirror, you can see what has to be seen. Check the pubic hair follicles for swellings, redness or itchiness. Then part the fleshy outer labia and, holding a magnifying mirror, move your fingers around, feeling and looking for the site and possible source of the trouble.

Examine any scars - such as those left by an episiotomy or tears - feel for any bumps, lumps or spots; check whether the anus is red and oozing, likewise the vaginal opening. Ring a special clinic if the perineum needs swabbing and professional examination.

Do not clean out the vagina before going for swabs and do not drink for three hours because urine must be concentrated.

Always be your own detective, the doctor has no time!

CHAPTER TEN

10 Clothing

A Brief History of Underwear

Only since the 1940s have women worn close-fitting knickers. Cotton, or silk if you were rich, were natural, breathing materials, soft enough for women to wear next to their skin. In the 1920s and 1930s, the French cami-knicker in silk, voile or very fine cotton lawn was loose with a crotch low enough not to get caught between labia or buttocks when sitting. Before that, Edwardian women wore longer pantaloons/bloomers secured at the waist with tie-strings and at the knees with pretty ribbons, all very loosely crotched and of cotton.

Victorian women wore these too, but because the crinoline gowns made bathroom/garden privy visits a near impossibility, they had wide open crotches which were very much easier for squatting on potties. Potties were positioned all over the home - in bedrooms, naturally, but also anterooms and small 'retiring rooms' in larger homes affording more privacy.

Beyond Victorian times open crotches were absolutely normal for underwear. Layers of petticoats and the long pantaloons were women's standard clothing, necessary for coping with life in cold, unheated homes. Open-crotched underwear and petticoats were seldom removed even in bed, so sexual access was also provided for.

What a long way we have 'progressed'! We cover up our perineum in gusseted, closed styles of underwear. We use cotton in all weights and colours and we use nylon/viscose/rayon to create patterned or see-through glimpses of flesh. Gussets of man-made materials, even those with a cotton inner fining inhibit air. From the sex industry many ordinary girls are now persuaded to wear thongs, a perineal disaster, so that tight jeans, leotards and trousers have no panty marks. Thongs are hard, seamed and capable of injury.

We may prefer a seamless gusset for comfort and we certainly no longer have the extended protection of long cotton petticoats, but do we have to wear underwear all the time? Do we really have to deny our perineums the air which their naturally open physiology requires?

We have very moist perineums and normal discharges. If we add on sweat to the natural moisture, we greatly encourage the spread of bacteria and fungus infestation. Think of the foot and toe fungal problems that have arisen since the advent of trainers and other types of running shoes, and of the upsurges of thrush and dermatitis since tights, leotards and leggings arrived.

These miserable health problems have arrived since the advent of antibiotics in the 1940s and modern clothing. Be user-friendly and remove your underwear when you are at home. Only buy 100 per cent cotton knickers, without that biting seam which some manufacturers sew on the crotch joins. Keep air flowing around your perineum at all times.

This then being the rule, if you want to stay genitally/sexually healthy, take a look at the clothes you wear for business, sports and hobbies to see how, in these unavoidable situations, you can still treat the perineum properly.

At Home/Work

HOME CLOTHES

- Keep warm with long body vests/T-shirts, slips/petticoats.
- Keep cool with longer cotton dresses in the summertime.
- Wear culottes or longer woollen skirts rather than trousers.
- Don't wear leotards.
- Go without underwear when convenient and comfortable.
- Wear cotton knickers, no thongs.

WORK CLOTHES

- Wear cotton knickers.
- Don't wear unbreathing tights which create moisture.
- Don't wear trousers; wear culottes in any natural cloth according to the season if your job requires this sort of clothing.
- Check the office chair: Is it propelling your knickers for six hours at a time up into the sensitive vulval skin? Shift your position every so often; take a soft feather cushion to sit on.
- Walk around frequently to aerate the perineum.
- Don't wear short skirts and cross your legs all the time.

Sports Activities

SWIMMING

Choose a clear water pool, not cloudy from chlorine; peer closely at its contents - any stringy, jelly-type substances floating about? Don't touch it! Likewise, if it is green, slimy and heavily used, especially by children, don't go near it. I've had two pools closed in my time and I've caught Gardnerella in a famous private members' pool! Trust nothing - examine it. If it seems OK. then swim, jacuzzi sensibly (for no more than seven minutes because of antiseptics in the hot water) and get out. Then:

- Shower straight away
- Dress and go to the cloakroom, fill the 500-ml bottle from your toilet bag, pass urine and then bottle wash the vagina and perineum to remove most of the chemicals found in pool water.

Sea-bathing can give you brain damage these days! Even if it is a quiet bay somewhere, check with locals that it isn't quiet because they all know the sewage outlet is there! Check out factory waste and all the other relevant environmental factors (the media is usually quite good at keeping us up to date on any hazards). Back at the guest house, clean out the vagina just to be on the safe side! Don't be tempted by the gleaming bidet! Bottle Wash properly!

Obviously, you have no choice but to wear a swimsuit. Rinse it thoroughly and change rather than let it dry on you. You may notice other women standing at the pool-side shower, their backs to you, fiddling away down the front of their swimsuit to clean the vulva! Quite right, too!

KEEP FIT, AEROBICS, WORKOUTS, GYMS

This is all about sweating! Elevated body temperatures give candida/thrush the green light for upsurging. Thrush loves heat and usually where there is heat, there is sweat. Pubic hair perspiration helps fungus embed itself in and between hair follicles. If attempts are made to cool down, the combination of non-porous leotard crotches, several leotards worn together, the exercise heat and the amount of time spent exercising will all conspire to cause sweating. Even after a shower it can still be some time before you cool down and stop sweating entirely.

Women with cystitis or thrush usually stop exercising because they just cannot manage it anymore, but some struggle on, further depleting their lowered immune system. I advise cystitis/thrush patients not to exercise until they are perfectly well again. Gyms can be addictive, two gentle work-outs a week or two good walks round the park are enough if you are well, too much if the perineum is unwell!

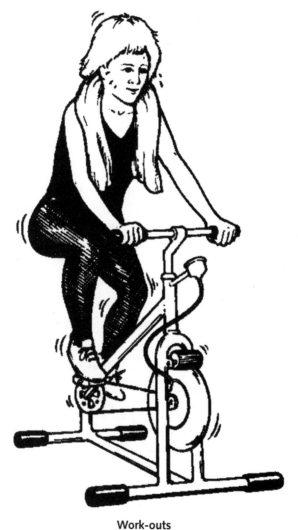

Work-outs

BALL GAMES

Same problems as for Aerobics, etc.

RIDING

Different problems, unless it is high summer when sweating is common. The basic difference is the bruising that occurs from the jodhpur/jean seam pounding into the vulva and a higher bladder bruising from bouncing in the saddle. An unusual symptom can be bleeding. It is blood from the bladder/urethra and is often unaccompanied by other symptoms like frequency or pain. Soreness and a feeling of heaviness in the pelvic region may or may not accompany spotting on underwear. Play detective: if you were fine until you took up riding - or any sport for that matter - stop for a while and see if your symptoms lessen/disappear.

Laundering

Obviously, clean underwear is important. Bacterial or fungal colonization in dripped discharge or urine from the previous day makes wearing knickers for more than one day a hazardous practice. Don't wear knickers in bed because air is essential at night. If you know your vulval skin reacts badly to all washing powders/liquids, then choose black, not blue, cotton underwear and boil it clean. This may mean frequent shopping for new pairs, because only washing powders/liquids remove the stains.

If such sensitivity is not a problem, then just wash your underwear along with the rest of your normal load. Machines rinse pretty well these days, but you could always give your underwear an extra hand rinse if desired.

Young women coming for counselling usually arrive these days in trousers. It shows me that they have not read the book properly or even that they are not taking Thrush and Cystitis seriously enough. They get strong words from me and are instructed to change their wardrobe for at least two months to monitor the change in the way the perineum feels. Symptoms for such women will at least include non-stop twingeing. It takes ten days for this to decrease or disappear once clothing is changed to skirts. It appears miraculous, it is not! It is acknowledging how the female perineum prefers to be which is cool and dry!

CHAPTER ELEVEN

11 Lifestyle

In this one word, lifestyle, lie most reasons for both sorts of cystitis - bacterial and non-bacterial. Everything written in this book so far supports this.

Lifestyle at home, work, in leisure-time pursuits must be discussed.

Until I began my work in 1971, a patient's involvement with her own cystitis was absolutely nil.

'Take the pills; take more pills; take the pills indefinitely.'

'It's a part of woman's lot!'

'You need tranquillizers, you're imagining it!'

'Have a baby, that works sometimes!'

'We'll dilate the urethra again!'

'You're hysterical!'

Frustration was enormous for patients and doctors; medical textbooks were impractical and unreadable and there was no literature for patients. Power and control now lie firmly in the hands of the patient.

The first light at the end of the tunnel was my Three-hour Management Procedure and the realization that passing water after intercourse helped. Suddenly the concept of a woman doing things at home to help herself began to emerge and we have not looked back to the bad old days. All around the UK (and other countries), hospitals, surgeries, nurses, teaching departments, magazines, TV and radio and countless ex-victims provide testimonials to the success of self-help methods for fighting cystitis.

Principles

All the major principles of self-help are now in place. Each new sufferer must simply get acquainted with them as quickly as possible. Cystitis will always exist, and will always erupt in those sensitive to it. Helplines, leaflets, media items, books, videos and personally spreading the word all help others learn about cystitis and to stop the threatened suicides which were all too common in the 1970's. One morning my phone rang at 9 a.m.; the caller was coping with her first ever attack beginning at 4.30 that morning! It was the earliest I had ever been contacted for advice on an attack (the previous record being three weeks, again after a first bout).

In the early years of my work, when material was not widely available and suffering was terrible, I ran a 24-hour help line; nowadays I get a bit annoyed if I am rung out of office hours, because so much other help is available. Friends can help you; the bookshop or library; the doctor's surgery; the pharmacy, so many sources of help are at hand. Of course, if any woman reading this book still needs counselling I will see her, but the message is to help yourself, using all the carefully researched and described rules laid out here. Don't think you know better than me and change basics. If I say a 500-ml bottle, I truly mean it; others have been tried and have failed for specific reasons.

If I say that three to five pints (60-100 fl.ozs) of water a day should be drunk, I mean it.

If I say wear skirts not trousers etc., I mean it!

Ignore, change or bend the rules and you will find out that I was right! Read, absorb and digest slowly and carefully.

Having said all this, I teach the principles and give plenty of additional help by examples. What I cannot be expected to account for are the thousands of habits and circumstances that millions of households practise.

Last autumn I lectured at a large hospital, from which a doctor referred a 'very difficult' patient to me in London. I can't tell the whole story, which included incorrectly taken urine samples that gave false results, job stress, HRT and a high sugar intake, but I will tell you of just one exchange I had with this woman:

'And you've bottle-washed after passing a stool, as I advised?'

'Absolutely, yes.'

'How often do your bowels open? Every day, every other day?'

'Oh, no! Every 13 days and it just seems to explode!'

No one, except someone with a severe bowel adhesion, goes that long and lives! Yet despite all the pills, liquids, etc., this had been her lot. What caused it? I found she'd had a severe addiction to sugar since childhood. Desperate, and now in her late thirties, she stopped sugar on my suggestion and, hey presto! her bowels now happily open without any help, every other day. My advice is always: bottle wash after passing a stool without fail. I would never have thought to account for a *13 day interval* between bowel movements! No wonder things still weren't right!

I will again say that Full Bottle Washing which is also called Procedure 1 in this section of the Encyclopaedia, is essential after any bowel movement, BEFORE ANY kind of sexual/digital activity, first thing in the morning AND last thing at night. It is meant for all teenage, adult and elderly women. Children must be carefully bathed every night.

Patient's Approach

The only acceptable changes in bottle washing, for instance, may be in patients who have disabilities such as Multiple Sclerosis, arthritis, paraplegia or the many other diseases or injuries that make one's movement or strength uncertain. But these changes should and can be designed to suit each individual.

I won't accept laziness or sloppiness when health is at stake. I like a patient who tries; if she is not quite sure about something, I will help to correct it. I won't accept sheer stupidity though:

'Well, why aren't you doing the bottle washing after every bowel movement?'

'Because it makes such a mess.'

'No it doesn't. How are you making it make a mess?'

'Well, you demonstrated it to me with your clothes in place. I always have to pull my skirts up and pull my knickers down when I'm on the toilet. I just can't do it like you!'

Of *course* I keep my clothes on for demonstrations!! I'm not undressing in front of other people! Of course, if it is for real, in my bathroom, I pull my knickers down and hold my skirt up, like everyone else!!

I hate cystitis on my own behalf and on all other victims' behalf, but my sympathy is limited. Individual diagnosis, and practical action is required to conquer your own cystitis. It is a battleground and I have come from the ranks to be the Commander. I fight and control, so must you.

Gynaecological Problems

These can include the gynaecologist! He or she may be disastrous, not spotting the problem in the first place, adding to the problem, or making things worse.

I saw a woman last year who took away with her a long list of ideas and suggestions. Nine months later she rang and, though her symptoms had improved, they had not gone entirely. We ran through my list and she had complied with everything except the first suggestion - to see a gynaecologist in London since her local ones had not found anything wrong. My hunches tend to be accurate. Having persuaded her, she came down to London and, within 40 minutes of seeing a gynaecologist there, a growth, now the size of a plum, had been discovered in the cervical canal. Urgent phone calls followed and she was admitted to hospital in her area, London being too distant. She is now improving.

Doctors and dentists are human, yet we put an abnormal amount of trust in them. Just because they have passed exams does not mean they are all-knowing.

Always get a second opinion, and even question test results closely. Practically every gynaecological problem can affect the bladder and urethra, which, after all, lie in close proximity to the uterus and vagina. There are many ways in which our reproductive organs can cause trouble in the bladder and urethra.

Retention of Urine before a period can cause cystitis, stinging and bloating, but thrush before a period is a matter of hormones and vaginal alkalinity. See to these and symptoms decline. For some the problems may be resolved by taking the contraceptive Pill, for others Evening Primrose Oil. Close attention to diet and exercise, and maybe a daily diuretic pill from the pharmacy may also help. An acid-based vaginal jelly inserted at night for a week encourages acidity rather than alkalinity. An alkaline vagina before a period helps thrush breed faster if it is present.

Pregnancy may stop or start cystitis. Urinary frequency is one of many features in early pregnancy whilst later on the opposite can be true for many women. A heavier vaginal discharge called Non-Infective Leucorrhea from increasing hormonal output can irritate the urethra. Hemorrhoids can cause cystitis by harbouring fecal bacteria in their crevices. The growing baby also affects bladder capacity meaning more short trips to the toilet!

Rest up when possible. Do a gentle vaginal bottle wash morning and night to clear out any irritating discharge regularly. A full bottle wash after a bowel movement cleans off the residue on hemorrhoids.

Childbirth can lead to cystitis (either bacterial or non-bacterial) while you are in hospital. Bacterial cystitis can come from catheterization, tearing, stitching, dirty commodes, bidets and toilet seats stained with blood and debris. Line the seat with toilet paper before using it. Carefully wash your perineum before actual delivery, if possible. Bottle wash daily in hospital to keep external stitching clean. Dry carefully and expose the perineum to plenty of air. Place pads underneath and let the vulva be exposed beneath your nightie or sheet.

Non-bacterial cystitis is usually caused by bruising during the baby's emergence. Rest, coolness and painkillers will all help after a few days. Any antiseptics known to cause cystitis must be avoided. Be firm: 'Don't swab me with any sort of antiseptic please. I have washed very carefully and antiseptics give me cystitis!'

Hemorrhoids and episiotomy scars are a common cause of cystitis after childbirth. Only daily Bottle Washing stops fecal germs harbouring or travelling to the urethral and vaginal openings.

Menopause/Hysterectomy often cause soreness, dryness, cystitis, stinging. Lowering hormone levels do not just make our faces wrinkle. They also make our urethras, vaginas and perineums wrinkle. It is called ageing, or atrophy. Skin gets thin, cracks and encourages bacterial growth. Sex is dry and miserable. Local creams, oral treatment, Red Clover from health-stores, patches or implants will help restore urethral, vaginal, perineal, sexual and bladder health.

Old Age is a major cause of cystitis. It is hormonal. Stiffening wrists, arms or necks prevent easy perineal cleaning. Commodes need daily cleaning and all the factors mentioned for the menopause apply, but even more so. Catheters and pads can cause soreness, bleeding and infection. Hormones can definitely be prescribed to older women. Doctors are happy now to prescribe them for most women over forty, but have not quite understood that they can help those over sixty. Red Clover is fine, too. Keep asking! If you are choosing a nursing home, ask to see the bathrooms, toilets and kitchen - never mind the lounge!

Ovarian Cysts if left untreated may cause symptoms throughout the reproductive organs and influence the urethra, causing stinging and frequency. Another sign of cysts may be a stiff back.

Polyps anywhere in the uterus, cervix or vagina can cause secondary stinging and cystitis. Polyps usually ooze and retain organisms which become a drippy discharge and affect the vulva and urethra.

Vaginal Thrush /Yeast can and does cause perineal soreness, irritation, urethral and bladder pain and also cystitis. If it is cyclical, use an acid-based vaginal jelly to increase vaginal acidity (which declines before a period). If it is present at other times, check:

- your sexual partner - is he a beer/alcohol drinker, a heavy sugar/cheese eater?
- your diet - do you eat a lot of cheese, cream, sugars, yeasts, chocolate, mushrooms, 'windy' foods, excessive bread, rice, potatoes? Do you drink a lot of alcohol or canned/cartonned drinks?
- your bedding - nylon, dacron, terylene duvets, nylon nighties or panties? Remember too, to keep cool - use cotton or other natural fibres wherever possible.
- your job - too hard, too energetic? Your work clothes too constricting/non-cotton? Are you sitting all the time? Is your energy depleted?
- illness - ME (viral fatigue), flu, HIV/AIDS, cancer and many other serious

illnesses, or just being tired and run-down, can all contribute to thrush.
- drugs - antibiotics, steroids, ulcer drugs, antacids?
- your hobbies - elevated body temperatures, leotards, swimming?
- your clothing - nylon underwear, tight skirts, jeans, leggings, corsets?
- Dental mercury depletes the immune system causing non-stop candida.

Remember:

- Keep cool; avoid sugar, certain drugs, certain clothes, men (for a while, anyway!); change jobs if you can, monitor your hobbies.
- Keep well and fresh, take oral and local anti-fungal treatments when you are hit by a big upsurge of yeast.
- Get those mercury fillings out safely and feel the immune system improve.

Erosions (cell overgrowth) of the cervix can cause soreness, frequency and/or cystitis. Symptoms like these and an exuding erosion require that it be removed. Symptoms should then cease. You might have to fight for a cautherisation since many doctors are inclined to want to leave it alone and if it has already gone into the cervical canal you may need a general anaesthetic. A second cauthery three months later might be needed, so press for checks.

All Vaginal Infections can cause secondary non-bacterial cystitis. Inflammation from Chlamydia, Gardnerella, Trichomonas, Myco ureaplasma and lots of other bacteria or parasites spreads out and on to the perineum. Urethral contact is quickly established and urethral nerves begin to react. Only a vaginal swab will disclose the specific vaginal infection and then the correctly sensitive antibiotic. Urinary symptoms will correspondingly decrease. Don't Bottle Wash for 12 to 15 hours before the swab is taken or the swab result will be negative.

Herpes can cause urinary stinging during an outbreak or even full-blown (non-bacterial) cystitis depending upon the site of the blisters. Read the literature on herpes and try to prevent it. Treat any outbreak instantly with one of the suggested medications. Lysine from any pharmacy - taken daily as a preventative, then more heavily if a blister appears - seems to be quite helpful in avoiding severe outbreaks. Stress levels from any source can activate this virus and its pain.

Thyroid/Endocrine malfunctions can cause bladder trouble. Other symptoms abound, but this book is about bladders. A really competent endocrinologist with many tests at his or her disposal can provide the best diagnostic and therapy results.

Surgery and Scarring negatively affect bladder and urethral tissue. Interference of any kind with nerve endings causes reactions such as twingeing, frequency, aching and feelings of heaviness.

Of all pelvic organs, the exceptional sensitivies of the urethral and bladder nerve endings make reactions possible at any time. Careless scalpel work or bruising of the bladder during surgery can result in a lot of misery for the patient. Scar tissue may adhere, blocking or obstructing the bladder so that it cannot work to full capacity. Prolapse surgery needs great skill and care - not a quick hitch and a few ill-placed stitches. Urethral and bladder dilatations scar forever eventually decreasing urethral and bladder function. Bacterial colonization is encouraged by weakened tissue defences.

Urological Conditions

URINARY LEAKING/INCONTINENCE.

There are many leaflets and much help available from continence advisers these days. They are fully trained nurses who have specialized in urinary care in order to help the huge numbers of women who suffer from leaking or varying degrees of incontinence. Ask at your doctor's surgery/local hospital for their help.

Leaking is more likely to occur in a woman who has experienced a difficult labour and has lost muscle tone on the perineum. The urethral sphincter valve (which lets urine out of the bladder) may also have stretched a bit, leaving a less tight seal when it is closed and the urethral opening may have distended a little also. There are good exercise books for strengthening the pelvic floor muscles but, once you get the hang of it, pulling up and tightening the perineum can be done sitting or standing with a minimum of fuss whenever you want.

Urinary dribbling or leaking when sneezing, laughing coughing or bending down happens because skin, muscles, ligaments, organs lose tension and support with age. HRT (if appropriate) can help, but nature and ageing are inexorable. **Slight weight gain** (even as little as three pounds) can make the difference between the urethral sphincter managing to 'hold' urine within the bladder or leaking if sneezing, bending or laughing. Heavy weight gain poses greater problems: no ageing bladder or urethral sphincter can withstand a great downward pressure, and incontinence garments may have to be worn.

Watching your weight starts in middle age, by sixty it may be too late! Keep the weight off, bowels regular and stay off sugars, fats, 'windy' foods, sweets, alcohol, etc. Exercise reasonably and tone up the perineum as often as possible. If the problem seems to be a prolapsed bladder, then get two opinions and good-quality scans. The uterus can sometimes by its own pressure relocate (prolapse) the bladder, in which case the uterus will have to be lifted away. Ask local nurses and women who may have had a prolapse operation, which surgeon's operative success rate is better than another's! If you don't like a surgeon's attitude, don't trust his or her operative skills either. We have all had enough of 'You'll be all right, my dear, next patient please.' Doctors should have to take courses in counselling skills these days before they are given their degree.

Urinary leaking can also be a sign of a very low-grade bacterial infection of the urethra and bladder. This is common in older, arthritic women who don't shower, bath or wash as they need to. I know of women in their eighties who bottle-wash twice a day (morning and bedtime) without any difficulties. Implement this simple cleaning procedure, paying special attention to soaping thoroughly between and around hemorrhoids and then rinsing off from the front with the bottle until all the soapiness has dropped off down the toilet. I lecture a lot to continence advisers and they swear by this routine. Disabled, injured, ill or incontinent patients have all stopped getting infections once taught bottle washing.

I have said nothing about urological problems such as stones, diverticuli, reflux, stenosis and more. Usually one visit to a urologist for a scan, x-ray or cystoscopy should reveal these sorts of problems. They are not everyday occurrences in general practice and because they are easily spotted with urological diagnosis, such conditions never come my way.

Men

I have also neglected men. Obviously men get far less cystitis than women because of the length of their urethral tube inside the penis and because anal bacteria have impossibly far to travel there, but sexual infections can cause urethritis, or prostatitis in later years. Anal homosexual intercourse and certain lifestyle causes such as heavy alcohol intake can also make for very miserable symptoms. Much in this book can also benefit any men who are in need of understanding and ideas. The main message, though, is use a condom, always take a thorough shower before any sex and cut down on alcohol/sugars. Myco bacteria live in your foreskin often causing NSU's. They transmit easily to any mouth during oral sex and into the vagina during intercourse!

In the Bathroom

Only three pieces of bathroom equipment are required for personal hygiene:

- A toilet and basin
- A bath/shower.

These are available absolutely everywhere. All homes from the humblest to the mightiest have these, so no excuses for smelling, please! Unfortunately, the perfect-shaped toilet hasn't yet been invented. It ought to be an inch longer from seat front to seat back than it is at present, so that we would all have a little more room in front for bottle washing, but it is all quite manageable as it is. Bidets are downright dangerous:

- They cause vaginitis and cystitis.
- They aren't plumbed far enough away from the wall for leg room as you *face* the taps, so fecal germs run towards the vulva.
- Temperature control is impossible before water hits the vulva.
- Water doesn't travel upwards and round the corner to the anal opening, and if it does it will only run downwards to the vagina again with all the fecal germs.
- A central spray is a bacterial blender, not a clean front-to-back flow.
- It is a 'luxury' item and few homes have them, thank goodness!
- Hospital bidets are never to be touched! Filthy!

Washing Sequences

Separate toilets create difficulties for bottle washers because they must walk back and forth. In every home there should be at least one and a sizeable basin in the same room.

Showers are cheaper and better than baths (in terms of the spread of bacteria), but so long as bottle washing is the prime washing procedure, a bath once a week is alright but do shower every day. Please finish by facing the shower, parting your legs and checking by feel that no soap or shower gel is trapped on the perineum or between the labia to irritate the rest of the day or night.

Moving house or staying away will involve differences in the new bathroom. Watch out for little things like the basin being so close to the toilet that you think you won't have to stand up to soap the anus. You do still have to stand up! Body positioning and gravity are always important. Perhaps you have succumbed to the sparkling blue bidet and now there are vaginal swabs showing Klebsiella on the cervix. Take the antibiotics and put a fern in the bidet!

Perhaps your cystitis starts every Sunday at your new boyfriend's home? Does the central heating stay on so that Bottle Washing is done in a warm bathroom? Or is it too cold to get out of bed to do it? Have you just bought a double bath for pre-sexual soaking - this is too hot, inflammatory and drying; sexual lubrication will be soaked away, though a lubricant gel could remedy this. Does the toilet get cleaned every day or does he share his house with some less-than-hygienic folk? Is the bathroom down stairs and through the kitchen where everyone else has congregated for a late evening supper! No matter the hurdles, anything stopping you Bottle Washing when you should, has to be corrected.

Changing Homes/Boyfriends/Diet/Job/Exams

HOMES

Stress! A house move, with all the cleaning, painting, drilling, gardening, entertaining, not to mention the money worries or discussions this entails, can negatively affect anyone's hormones for a couple of months. Try a holiday - no money left? Try the well-woman clinic, it's cheaper! If it is not hormones it may be dehydration, irregular liquid intake when you actually need more at this time because of increased physical activity. Perhaps you have celebrated too well! Which rules have you bent, broken or neglected that kept cystitis at bay before?

BOYFRIENDS

All sorts, extra-marital as well. Is the bathroom unsuitable? Are you Bottle Washing before sex? Does he insist that you have some wine too? Has a new need for contraception arisen? Does using this new sort coincide with the first sign of twingeing? Is he uncircumcised and not really cleaning the foreskin? Does he shower properly? Does he take you swimming, drinking, curry-eating, chilli-eating? Does he take you climbing, driving, diving. Anything to chafe, irritate, dehydrate? Does he have new (for you) or unusual sexual habits? Does he want to use sex toys analy and then vaginally? What is his job - does he use chemicals, building materials, sit at a desk and have long nails? Check his underwear and towels for fecal staining! The possibilities are endless and highly individual. Look to all these factors and more to find what has triggered your cystitis.

DIET

All sorts of social factors lead to dietary changes. Perhaps you have decided to become a vegetarian? Veggie foods cause bloating and farting, with the accompanying dangers of wind-borne expulsion of fecal germs. Have you gone to live abroad? Wherever it is, from New York to Addis Ababa, foods and liquids will be different enough to cause problems. Are diarrhoea or loose stools now a daily hazard? Maybe too much garlic in each meal is causing looser stools, or drinking a different kind of tea. Perhaps you are suddenly eating more sugar, or are dehydrated, or comfort eating because of boredom. Look for the differences, experiment and then institute changes back to the old, safe ways. Constipated? Have you started eating meat, rice or eggs every night? Are you favouring brewed coffee or pure orange juice nowadays for breakfast after that gourmet break in Bruges? Snacking on chocolate or fruit gums?

JOB

Who would think that daily work could influence the urethra and bladder! Ask yourself:

First Question - did cystitis coincide with a career move, a change of office, a change of job, a change of boss, starting shift work? Are the toilets far away and you now 'hold it'?

Second Question - If so, how does this affect the primary causes of bacterial/non-bacterial cystitis (see below).

You may be able to pinpoint the exact date on which symptoms began, or it may take longer before becoming aware that 'something isn't right'. Once an idea forms and is proved by urine and vaginal samples, put the circumstances right and see if it happens again.

Is it Bacterial Cystitis?

Do you now have to catch an earlier train, which means that instead of bowels opening before leaving, you have to wait until arriving at work? Bottle Washing routines need careful, practical re-alignment (see Chapter 5).

Shift-work upsets some women's sensitive bodies. Be prepared to give it up if necessary - you may earn less but you will feel better. Did you forget to pack the bottle for a business trip? In its absence what was used - a mug? If so, there was probably not enough water to get rid of all the soap! Better to bring up a bottle from the bar, 500 ml or 2 x 300 ml. Try to think of *any possible* disturbance to your routine. It may be significant enough to have caused a bout of bacterial cystitis.

Is it Non-bacterial?

Is the new office chair pressuring the urethra from underneath and your weight pressing from above all day long? Blood vessels constrict, then expand, creating a slight swelling as they do so. Five days a week of this may mean a distinctly uncomfortable bladder by Friday night. Have the guys propelled you each lunchtime into the new wine bar for a quick drink, or two, or three on Fridays? Come 5 p.m. and dehydration may be causing twingeing. Drink mineral water, not alcohol. Is the person who cleans the cloakroom off sick? Always line the seat and sit comfortably. Is the boss too demanding upon your time/energy!?

Remember to drink and void at regular intervals.

EXAMS

Varying degrees of stress result in changes to our behaviour. Reading all day in the library in jeans/other uncomfortable clothing produces the same problems as office staff can encounter. Relaxing in the pub afterwards just adds insult to the day's inertia and lack of dietary care. Thrush may upsurge too, from the lack of air to perineal skin and too many chocolate bars for energy! Perhaps your underwear isn't being changed or washed properly and ageing mucous is starting to harbour bacteria, or maybe rinsing is less than satisfactory. If you are tired, thrush can upsurge and an early signal may be urethral twingeing. Pace yourself as best you can with regular meals and drinks, regular sleep, and a few hours to relax properly between study sessions. Take exams wearing skirts not jeans, the vulva will benefit, not bruise.

HOLIDAYS

How many of us have had a much-needed, well-earned holiday ruined by cystitis or vaginitis of some sort?

The main thing is to step *up* the rules, *not* think, 'it'll be fine, I'm on holiday!' A holiday is a huge hazard, since too much of everything that can cause cystitis - sex, sun, swimming, heat/ cold, alcohol, food, perhaps even stress - is the norm. Keep following all the rules, and have a great time. Stick a toothbrush in your bottle-wash bottle to stop the cleaners taking it away!

A Final Word

In the fight against cystitis, self-diagnosis by taking a look at your lifestyle is paramount. Reading this book and searching for clues are pre-requisites to success once urine sample results have accumulated and been understood. So much is caused unwittingly by women themselves that, given much needed understanding and information it is perfectly possible to reduce and eradicate cystitis without medical interference.

Good luck!

Further Interest

Patients Against Mercury Amalgams (and other dental practices) has a large Compendium full of help for discovering more about mercury poisoning but mailing to the States is prohibitive. Please go into www.google.com and check out the DAMS site for Defense Against Mercury Syndrome. They have State-wide co-ordinators and a great newsletter.

BOOK TWO

Sexual Cystitis

CHAPTER 1

1 Basics

Cystitis is just a symptom of something else wrong. Find the something else wrong and you stand an excellent chance of stopping the cystitis. Many more women than men get cystitis and four out of five women will experience it at some stage in their lives. It can start literally at any time from birth to death for an infinite number of reasons but there are some points in the female's cycle when she would appear to be more at risk. These points are:

1. Childhood
2. Puberty
3. Onset of regular sexual relations
4. Pregnancy
5. Childbirth
6. Menopause
7. Hysterectomy
8. Old age

In Sexual Cystitis, I propose to look in great detail at sexual causes. Until their first-ever attack many women, especially young ones, don't even know the condition exists. Then they panic.

The symptoms of cystitis/urinary tract infection are,

1. Pain on passing urine
2. Frequency of passing urine
3. Fever
4. Backache
5. Nausea

Not everyone experiences all these symptoms. You can have only two or three of them, in any order or any severity from just nuisance value through to screaming agony. Young sufferers go to the doctor fast but older ones will learn to use a combination of self-help and medical help. Over many years, countless magazines and newspaper articles, television and radio programmes have promoted my ideas on prevention and management of urinary problems. Leaflets, lectures and my websites now push hospitals and health-centre doctors to recommend the values and virtues of managing cystitis preventively rather than by senseless operations and needless repeat antibiotics.

Just because your cystoscopy (bladder and urethral examination under anaesthetic) shows inflammation, don't run away thinking that this in itself is an illness or an answer. You have yet to discover its cause! IVPs (intravenous pyelogram - X-ray) of the kidneys, bladder and urethra are also usually negative for most women with cystitis.

MSUs (mid-stream urine samples) are of the utmost importance and must be taken for proper analysis. Whatever the result, it is vital to know it and it is the first major clue for any line of investigation.

Vaginal and cervical swabs are *always* a good idea. Insist on having them and on knowing the result. A swab looks for bacteria; a Smear/Pap test looks for abnormal or cancerous cells. Gynaecological interest in vaginal health is low and patients deserve better treatment in this area.

Refuse urological operations like urethral dilations unless at least one other urologist agrees with the first one and they both have the same foolproof medical reason for wanting to stretch your urethra and bladder.

Dilations scar the linings of the bladder and urethra, muscle strength is lost on the scar and failure rate is high. No, you do not have a narrowed urethra unless you are elderly and need hormone replacement therapy.

There is just no medical excuse for operating on a cystitis patient when one kidney X-ray and one cystoscopy have both come up negative. Common sense is all!

It is far better to ask a straightforward question: When did your cystitis start?

If it started, say, when you were seventeen years old, it's safe to assume that your bladder worked perfectly well up to then, therefore nothing of a serious nature can be causing the cystitis and it's the same at any age.

Medical and patient frustration can be acute and until my work began, many women were put on lengthy tranquillisers. You really aren't alone: millions of women everywhere get cystitis and know just what you're going through. Frustration comes from lack of knowledge. There's plenty of knowledge available these days. So now you're going to learn.

Having found my work, have you discussed it with your doctor? Take more responsibility for your own health and remove some of his workload because self help is the best alternative to sitting regularly in the waiting room.

Medical education is a continuous process and a good doctor learns from medical magazines, patient's reports, laboratory reports, drug company representatives, courses, medical papers and books. Cystitis is one of the commonest female complaints and your doctor will be very thankful to have new information on it. Show this book.

From a total lack of sex education in my day, most schools now give courses but hygiene before intercourse is hardly mentioned. Emphasis remains on how it happens and how to prevent unwanted pregnancy. Condoms, vaginal sponges, spermicidal gels, creams, foams and morning-after pills are easily obtained and regular sexual activity can be catered for by going on the Pill at an early age whether or not parents know. Homosexuality has become open and such knowledge reaches gullible, receptive teenagers.

Inner-city schooling and parenting creates inner-city offspring - streetwise and sexually strident. Drugs and porn encourage and stimulate the shyest to indulge in sexual activities to 'try it out'.

This is sex education; make no mistake about it. Sex education is no longer confined to curricular or parental guidance over the dishwashing or at eleven o'clock on Tuesday morning after history! Television, films and advertising are very heavily involved but they never ever show pre-sex **hygiene**!!

Dr Henry Ritter, an American MD, writing in his book *From Man to Man* says, 'Parents have an obligation *to learn* how to play their roles as the primary sex educators.'

It isn't enough to feed, clothe, love and house your children. You must set standards, give guidance, lay down right and wrong and make sure that your children know about their own bodies and how humanity procreates.

Laugh if you must, explain why you've laughed, put your arms around their shoulders for a reassuring hug and then collect yourself ready to give straight answers to sexual inquisitiveness.

Years ago, my son reckoned he and his friends knew all about sex. "We all know the names - it's just we've no idea where they all go"! He said seriously. I roared and roared with laughter at the image of sixteen little boys whispering inaccurate settings of the testicles and womb! After informing him correctly I finished with the guarded advice to confine his knowledge to the S-E-X class and that really sex talk was best done within a confidential atmosphere. Not during assembly, for instance, just as talk of cricket or baseball in a music appreciation class is out of place. In other words, there's a time and a place for everything in life. Life has moved on from here because sex is a commonplace public subject now and it's a pity.

My sex life didn't begin until late courtship and engagement. It was not orgasmic or fulfilling - no early sex is. From the third day of my honeymoon I was out of sexual action because of cystitis. The next five years of intense attacks every three to four weeks and lasting two to three weeks meant an all-consuming existence of pain, incontinence, operations, antibiotics, vaginal thrush, examinations, and also three periods of six months each without sex, on doctor's orders. There was terrible fear, too. Fear of the next attack and the ensuing sexual deprivation, the rows, the distress and, of course, the physical symptoms to which one never became accustomed. They were just as terrible each time. Don't be fooled by anyone who proclaims cystitis an inconvenience. This problem can devastate a perfectly good marriage and wreck a career. My problem was utter ignorance about hygiene.

Sexual bonding in early marriage is seldom mentioned but all important. Don't put the office first and leave half an hour at midnight for a swift hump! You and your partner deserve better. Good sex takes thought, energy, weekends off and lots of love. Frequent casual sex sets fake standards, yardsticks and expectations. It can make bonding with someone really special very much harder later on, and make the habit of sleeping around difficult to break or refuse.

Sexual diseases have rapidly increased; sleep casually and you sleep uneasily. Bear in mind the dangers of ill health, unhappiness, embarrassment and loss of trust.

Determination of many parents to be seen 'not interfering' has made me equally determined to watch over my children's future marriages; to actively open doors before and during those marriages where they can seek detailed, confidential and intimate help. I believe that we must build up family units again, educate and love children, open lines of learning, talk pleasantly to one another, and have frequent, happy sexual intercourse, it's good for you!

Dear Angela,

I just thought I would write to you about my twenty-eight years of married life. I read one of your books about three years ago and lent it to a friend but never got it back. I think you could write a book about me as my surgeon has often told me to write one.

I was watching Breakfast Television this morning sitting on a bucket for one and a half hours, as I do most mornings because my toilet is upstairs and I can not get to it in time, when you came on the screen.

I started off with cystitis straight after my marriage. I was at the doctor's every three to four weeks getting tablets. My husband had to take some as well and we were unable to have sex for a week. I had a baby one year after our marriage and then cystitis carried on every three to four weeks and I carried on taking tablets.

I went back to the doctor and he said that I should take the Pill to stop it, but it didn't. I didn't get it quite so often but I still suffered terribly.

Tests, cystitis, biopsies, fourteen catheters, bladder washouts where I had to lay on my back for three days and have nitrate pumped into my bladder, where all the stuff used to come out in great big lumps with blood on it like a kettle that got scaled up, up to thirty-six bottles! The pain was unbearable sometimes but it had to be done. I also had a hysterectomy six years ago.

I have had three nervous breakdowns from 1982-83 then 1985-86. I was in hospital from 17 November until 11 February 1986. I have just got over that and I am now waiting to go into hospital again under a top surgeon to have my bladder taken out and a plastic bag installed. What else he is going to find I do not know as I am in so much pain. I really have suffered. I am told that I am a young looking fifty-years.

I have just retired after sixteen years because of ill health. I receive some pension. My husband has also lost his job at fifty-two years old. My daughter gets married on 7 September and my own marriage has just about ended.

With all the other things I have to do, I also have to look after my mother who is on tablets and is like a walking zombie, I am nearly going round the bend with worry over the operation. I have just about had enough, as your body can only stand so much.

I hope you don't mind me writing to you to tell you about everything, I don't think anyone else could have suffered so much and still look so good. It is a wonder that I am not as grey as a badger.

I can't sit down very well so I am always doing housework, and I go dancing. I can't go swimming, biking, or walk very far as I am always wet through and I have to wear padding to stop it coming through my clothes.

I hope for a bed anytime after next week as the surgeon was fully booked up in March and April. When I went to see him, I asked, 'What am I going to do for another eight weeks?' He said' Just keep wearing the padding and weeing'. I said, 'Great, I've been doing that for nine years.'

So there is my story, but there is a lot more to it besides - like riding in a car, weeing in bags and baby pads! Then stopping at garages to throw it away because there are no toilets on motorways. I have always gone behind trees otherwise.

I hope you don't mind me writing to you, but I have always wanted to see you and I did this morning, which I enjoyed very much.

Mrs S.Y. Humberside.

I have written Sexual Cystitis precisely to help Mrs S.Y. and millions of other young women. Marriages fail and sexual unhappiness occurs for an infinite number of reasons. I can help all women to enjoy better sexual health, but, only if you follow my routines properly.

Let me tell you a thing or two you may not have known about sexual health.

CHAPTER 2

2 The Vagina and Other Organs

We almost *abuse* the vagina today because contraceptives have changed its role forever. Originally it mostly facilitated fertilization of eggs and babies from the warm womb to the cold room but now look what it has to put up with! Repetitive sexual intercourse ad infinitum!

Every time that a penis is inserted, surrounding tubes and organs in the female have to make space for it, not so for the penis, being an external organ

Several sex sessions a week can initiate all sorts of bodily rebellions; tight, swollen breasts that hurt and need a larger bra, tiredness that upsets a day's work, tetchy moods, changes in urinary output, sore skin and cystitis.

Expectation of intercourse is now a social habit and women are expected to be sexually active from an early age, especially by their peers and boyfriends. Young men can have a prodigious output of erections and orgasms and have no hesitation in finding a freely available vagina, protected against pregnancy. There are so many about these days.

The freely available vagina, protected against pregnancy, is much more willing than ever before in history. Good contraception and ready abortion, if mistakes occur, give every woman the freedom to be willing, if she wants. She does want. Women now *want* almost as much as the men! Suddenly, after all these centuries of human existence, the vagina has become over-active. Holidays, central heating and more money mean more time for relaxing and sex.

Sensual clothes, erotic dancing, word of mouth, magazines and music all tell her she can. She can have intercourse whenever, wherever and with whom so ever it pleases her. Mother no longer says, 'Wait till you're married.' This is a major human biological revolution - early and repeated use of the simple birth canal solely for pleasure. Where will such activity lead?

We know it leads to more cancer of the cervix and to infections, but will it in tens of thousands of years' time lead to biological reproductive changes. It can lead to death! HIV Aids is an outcome of penetrative misuse of anus and lower bowel. These facilitate excretion of waste body products and poisons, not penile intercourse in either sex.

Reproductive organs became weakened by successive childbirth and weakened mothers had lower life expectancy leaving families uncared for. The idea of having several wives per husband was sensible. It gave each wife less daily work and with each pregnancy, lactation usually meant no sex either. Prostitution also had its uses - wives were less used for sexual pleasure but the life of the prostitute was often short!

Even from this very brief look at history, too much sex may seem detrimental to women's health, just as imitating men by wearing jeans and trousers is not good for vulval health. The body will at some point say, no!

Previous generations have spent their youth *without* sexual permissiveness. Wars took away most active sexual years and shortage of money meant less leisure for sexual activity. This has rapidly changed with contraception. But at the end of life modern science has moved ahead and antibiotics, diuretics and ventilators often prolong unnecessary suffering. Women now live a very long time but gynaecological care for elderly women may be poor.

Effective lifelong gynaecological care matters now because of increased sexual expectations and longevity so let's remind ourselves of the necessities for sexual activity.

Vagina

The Vagina in a child or a virgin is flat with all the sides touching. Upon losing virginity, it opens up to become a round tunnel. This tunnel or passage has the cervix at the top and the vulva at the bottom.

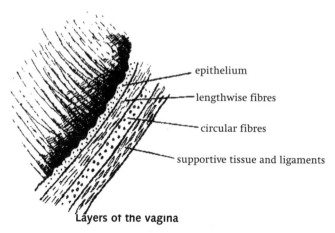

epithelium

lengthwise fibres

circular fibres

supportive tissue and ligaments

Layers of the vagina

It needs to be extremely elastic so its walls are muscular and fibrous. The skin that you can touch in the vagina is called the epithelium and has several layers before the fibre/muscle sections begin. Epithelial surface is moist and constantly shedding itself in the form of cells which also carry a number of other things with them like glycogen, lactobacilli and hormones, particularly estrogen.

If you have enough lactobacilli, the vaginal pH (levels of acidity and alkalinity) stays at around 4.5 - mildly acidic - and fends off most low bacterial and fungal invasions like thrush (Yeast infection). In children, before puberty, there's no glycogen and no lactobacilli making the vaginal pH around 7.0-7.5 and alkaline. Glycogen decreases after menopause with a corresponding drop in lactobacilli and acidity making the vagina alkaline again.

Beyond the circular muscle fibres at the outer layers of the vagina are layers of supportive skin tissue and ligaments to hold tissues in place. The major blood vessel is the vaginal artery, supplying blood to the vaginal area, and used blood is carried away from the area by branches and trunk of the iliac vein. The whole lower pelvic area, most particularly the vulva and its openings, is heavily supplied with tiny blood vessels and nerve endings for sexual excitement, reproductive functions, and oxygenation which provides strength for muscular activity during labour.

Hymen

The Hymen, at the lower end of the vagina, is a fibrous area of tissue mainly there to protect children and young girls from infections. It is usually broken easily enough by penile penetration, but in some girls can be too tough and needs surgical help to break. Some hymens are too elastic and can be nicked or split during intercourse only to mend again. Such hymens may finally rupture during childbirth but usually intercourse itself is sufficiently sore to need careful surgery. A hymen, if there's just too much of it, can limit the flow of menstrual blood and be responsible for low pain and swelling, so any girl starting periods and incapacitated by them should, for this and other reasons, be taken to a gynaecologist. I once read somewhere that virginity is the only object to become useful once you've lost it!

Vulva

The Vulva is the medical name given to the front area incorporating urethral and vaginal openings. It is rich in blood vessels, having arteries and veins interconnecting all over the place. The vulva has numerous lymph glands connecting down both its sides and supremely sensitive nerve supplies run from the clitoris right along to the anal opening.

Because both openings in the vulva lie so near to one another, they can frequently affect one another. Internally also they are closely situated.

Cervix

The Cervix is up at the top of the vagina. It should be thought of really as the end of the uterus not the end of the vagina. Part fibre, part muscle, the cervix has tremendous reserves of strength and elasticity for pushing the baby out. Around ovulation, due to cyclical hormonal changes, a mucous membrane manufactures and holds a little plug of liquid. This liquid lines the cervical canal and is additional nourishment for travelling sperm when ejected in intercourse. It is alkaline and full of carbohydrate to encourage sperm on their amazing journey upwards to the Fallopian tubes and ripe eggs.

Near one part of the cervix, there is only about half an inch distance between it and the ureters leading down into the bladder so that when a penis is introduced, its thrusting affects all organs nearby. Thicker surrounding tissue is there to help reduce internal bruising.

This padding is caused not only by eating and drinking sufficiently for a reasonable weight, its amount is also dictated by hormone activity. Estrogens and progestogens play a major part in the workings of the reproductive system and will be dealt with later on. Through the centre of the cervix runs a canal from the uterus which carries menstrual blood and unfertilised eggs.

Uterus/Womb

The Uterus/Womb is about three and a half inches long and in most women tilts forward so that it lies over the top of the bladder. It has muscle, about one inch thick. This muscle stretches with the developing fetus and then after birth sinks back, although floppier. Uterine width is about two and a half inches but this can vary greatly and its length is about three inches. It is extremely strong and flexible, and exercising it back to shape after birth is greatly recommended.

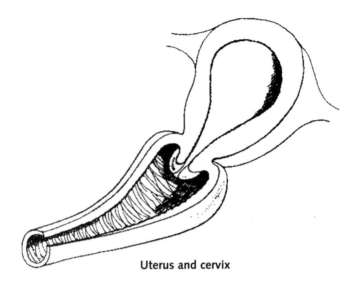

Uterus and cervix

Endometrium

The uterus has a lining called the endometrium, a brilliant piece of organisation on nature's part. This lining is constantly growing and discarding. It consists of rich blood, oozing out of blood vessels in uterine walls, which drops off every month from puberty to menopause. If there is no period bleed, an egg may have been fertilised or, there may be an underlying condition requiring investigation or in later life it may be onset of menopause.

Cervix / Fallopian Tubes

The Uterus has an upside down pear-shape, the stalk being the cervix and the flat fleshy part being the top. The top of the uterus contains two tubes called the Fallopian tubes in which swimming sperms encounter eggs ready for fertilisation. Eggs come from both of the two ovaries, which manufactured them many years in advance and now expel a small number each monthly cycle. Unfertilized eggs continue on from the Fallopian tubes into the uterus, where they get washed out of the body in each monthly bleed.

Pelvic Floor Muscles

The Pelvic Floor Muscles as you can see from the diagram, are a web-like network of incredible strength. They literally stop your internal organs from falling out. It you lose some of their strength, as after childbirth, there may be great nuisance effects of poor bladder control, bowel control or lowering of the uterus called prolapse. Regular lifelong exercises will maintain and regain their strength. Each and every day of your life when you pull up, push down, push out, sit in a chair, walk, etc., this network of muscles is at work commanded by the trillions of nerve endings that connect, through the spinal column, into bigger ones within the brain.

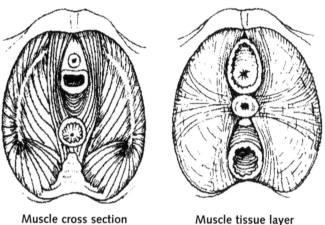

Muscle cross section   **Muscle tissue layer**

They, in turn, are protected by another layer of supportive smoother fibre and finer muscle.

Feces

It is worth understanding how our body digests the food we eat, because the bacteria controlling digestion and present in feces are the very ones causing so much sexual cystitis.

Acids, enzymes and bacteria work on the molecules of what was once delicious food and drink, but is becoming a brown emulsified mess. These molecules become so small that they can actually be absorbed through the lining of the duodenum and small intestine into the bloodstream where they deliver energy and nutrients. Unnecessary molecules continue into the large intestine ready for excretion.

Emulsified waste reforms into the shape of the colon becoming feces varying in width, length and shape according to what food or drugs you have eaten.

Whether liquid or hard, they absolutely teem with germs. Inside the bowel they are quite harmless, but outside they are able to travel to the urethral opening causing cystitis if it is a short journey.

Urethra

The urethral opening lies between the clitoris and vagina. The clitoris is the sensitive gland helping sexual arousal in foreplay. From its opening on the perineum, the urethral tube, or urethra, rises one and a half inches into the bladder and is lined with layers of epithelial cells known as the Epithelium.

The back wall of the urethra lies extremely close to the front wall of the vagina and consequently anything inserted into the vagina temporarily displaces, flattens or massages urethral walls whilst it's there.

Bladder

The top end of the urethra leads up into the bladder which receives waste body fluids. When two or three hundred millilitres of urine have accumulated, the bladder sends out signals that it wants to empty. Pelvic floor muscles loosen, and muscle contractions allow urine to escape down the urethra and out into the toilet pan.

Bladder muscular expansion and contraction works according to kidney output and is extremely sensitive. These muscles are covered by a rough mucous membrane that becomes much smoother and stronger near the internal end of the urethra known as the Trigone. This acts like the strengthened base of a bowl in order to bear the weight and pressure of gathering urine. Part of the bladder lies very close to the front walls of the womb and the bottom part lies directly on the front part of the cervix.

Ureters

In the top of the bladder are two openings which each lead into a ureter. Each ureter is about ten inches long and has a one-way valve at the bottom end allowing collected droplets of urine to pass just one way - downwards into the bladder. At their higher end, they become a renal pelvis which further enlarges into a kidney.

Kidneys

We each have two kidneys about the size of a medium cupped hand. They are an inch to an inch and a half thick, measure about four and a half inches from top to bottom and maybe two and a half inches wide. Without kidneys, or at least one, we would die. Kidney disease can therefore be life-threatening and was before antibiotics stopped rising bladder infections in the 1940's.

Each kidney's blood supply is inter-connected by the main artery and vein of the body. (Arteries carry blood to organs from the heart, and veins carry it away from organs back to the heart.) The artery that branches out of the big main body artery, or Aorta, is called the Renal artery and the vein that branches off the big main body vein into the kidneys is called the Inferior Vena Cava.

Renal arteries carry about fifteen continuously flowing gallons of blood an hour into each kidney and the Inferior Vena Cava carries it all out again. In that blood is carried all the minerals, salts, proteins, amino acids, vitamins and fats that our small intestines absorbed into their walls and on into the bloodstream.

So here is the big link up with what we eat and drink. An astonishing number of functions are performed by each kidney. The renal artery branches out into estuaries of finer arteries called capillaries. Estuaries are enclosed in capsules, Bowman's Capsules named after their discoverer. Each capsule collects water out of the blood and disperses it into a narrow tube called a renal tubule. Water is condensed into an even smaller, stronger amount which passes into other tubules sending the newly formed urine into the renal pelvis and down either ureter. When enough urine collects in them, sphincter valves open to allow urine into the bladder.

Urine

Urine is basically made of waste proteins called urea, but there is also some salt, body acids from digestion, uric acid, some fat, and water. Waste particles of carbohydrates and fats finally leave the body as carbon dioxide which our lungs breathe out, and not via the urine.

Normal yellow urine comes from urochrome; other variations in colour are influenced by the amount of liquid we have drunk. Drink too little and urine is more acid and browner in colour, drink a lot and it is much paler and doesn't sting.

Normal urine is slightly acid, but acidity levels can be varied by our daily liquid consumption. If protein is shown in a urine test it indicates a possible infection. If sugar is found in urine it may mean the bloodstream has been overloaded with a heavy sugar intake or it could also mean you are diabetic and have an insulin disorder.

Urine samples are taken for aiding the correct diagnosis of many illnesses and are as important as blood samples.

Pituitary Gland

The pituitary gland lies in the base of the brain reacting to the amount of water currently in the bloodstream. This organ is responsible for releasing a special anti-diuretic hormone. A diuretic substance makes you pass lots of urine, an *anti*diuretic *restricts* the amount you pass. This anti-diuretic hormone reduces urinary excretion by persuading the renal tubules not to discard water from the bloodstream but to hold on to it, so we bloat. The Pituitary gland is also the seat of sexuality and links up to infrequent urination during pre-menstrual tension.

There is much interlinking of systems within all renal functions and progress in understanding is still continuing.

I have given slightly more information in these descriptions of reproductive and renal organs than elsewhere because I do feel that we, as patients, need to upgrade our knowledge in order to help ourselves. If you need to get to grips with cystitis, it is important to understand something of gynaecological and urinary backgrounds.

PART ONE

Preparation For Intercourse

CHAPTER THREE

3 Sizes and Scars

Preparation for intercourse should involve both partners. We haven't discussed male internal organs because cystitis is overwhelmingly a female problem, but Non Specific Urethritis, Prostatitis, and other nasty diseases are more likely problems for men and transmittable.

Men

Without boring ourselves into madness, we must by now all know that his spermatozoa - sperm - are ejaculated all round and over the cervix during orgasm.

These millions of sperms swim through the cervical canal into the uterus and up into the Fallopian tubes where just one sperm impregnates and fertilises one egg. The egg can remain as one or divide up for twins, triplets, quads etc., passing down into the uterus for nine months.

Size and Shape

Male genitalia are not identical in shape, size or feel. A young man's penis may be too thin to fully pleasure a woman in her thirties after two or three children; it may be almost too hard when fully erect for a younger woman's comfort. Older men soften up somewhat and become more comfortable to bear during thrusting. Several sorts of dysfunction afflict the penis including failure to achieve a satisfactory erection. This can be a total non-starter, too soft or fail to maintain the erection. Orgasm can be too quick as in premature ejaculation or not even happen at all. Penile presentation can be crooked, bent to one side or have the rarer Peyronies Disease where it curls up like a pig's tail needing surgery. Men are not forthcoming about penile problems and women usually have either a shock on the first outing or a long battle with a reluctant husband unwilling to seek help as necessary! There is lots of help these days including herbal viagra and prescribable Viagra, sexual dysfunction clinics, surgery and many good books with information.

The majority of short men mate with short women, tall men with tall women and all the variations of size in between. A short woman, say five feet tall would, even with a good elastic vagina, be most unlikely to have comfortable intercourse with a man six foot two, and vice versa a short man to a tall woman. Penile size is important in love-making either causing or preventing sexual bruising and cystitis.

Foreskins

Foreskins vary tremendously. Heavy ones may prevent smooth vaginal entry and also harbour germs which transmit to the cervix. Persuade him to see a really good genito-urinary specialist and explain the sexual situation so that swabs of the mucous under the foreskin can be taken and analysed. Thin foreskins are far easier to clean inside and out and harbour fewer bacterial colonies. Condoms are the cleanest and most effective way of preventing sexual illness. Every woman should carry one, every man should carry several and they should be put on before ANY sexual contact starts.

Circumcision

A circumcised man can be two things to two women. One woman can revel in the firmness and cleanness of his thrusts in and out of her vagina but a tighter vagina could be bruised by that same firmness and rigidity.

I am a believer in male circumcision. There is new scientific evidence showing clearly that not only is AIDS less prevalent in circumcised societies but sexual diseases also. Foreskins harbour infections and mothers do not teach boys effective washing procedures. Men tend not use enough toilet paper. Scrunching it up fails to collect fecal residue efficiently, and so when the penis rests inside soiled underwear, fecal residue transfers to it. Then this can transfer to a vagina! Check on his underwear, provide pale-colored towels and then confront him!

Fingers

Fingernails are good indicators of careful hygiene. Look at his hands and nails, any ingrained dirt? Jagged? too long? Balance this with the job he does: you can't expect a motor mechanic to look as though he was the chairman of the Stock Exchange. The desk-bound man cannot afford to be proud either since he is often too thoughtless or lazy to wash after work at the office when he's arrived home, having read the paper and opened the train doors that everyone else touches.

One man always washed his hands in the washroom before coming home but oils from his job as a rig supervisor and site lecturer needed a second removal effort at home. So he reached for the washing up liquid *and* the heavy duty Swarfega every night. All his wife's urine results were negative over the seventeen years of her marriage, which had been blighted with cystitis. Her husband had always worked in the oil industry and they always had plenty of foreplay - a feature they both loved. The oils and oil removers were ingrained on his hands. He wasn't skin sensitive but she was.

Women
Hymen /Virginity

Not all hymens break easily at the first attempt at intercourse. With such natural apprehension and maybe the awkwardness of failure on first efforts, try again after a few hours with two or three strong painkillers and a good dollop of lubricating jelly from any pharmacy. If this and other attempts prove unrewarding and miserable, it's no good carrying on, so go to a gynaecologist.

Surgical removal should leave clean edges or jagged flaps will make intercourse sore and bloody with infections causing cystitis and misery so seek help quickly.

Thinly padded vaginal epithelial lining is easily traumatized by sex. Women beneath the hundred and twelve pound weight mark (eight stone), or anorexics, may suffer regular misery. Lubrication is poor and toleration of intercourse low. Vaginal soreness rapidly affects equally thin urethral muscles and fibres lying right in front of the vagina.

Vagina

Capable of great elasticity, its length from entrance to cervix doesn't alter in intercourse nearly as much as the width. If there is a length problem in any given sexual partnership the cervix is just going to be badly battered at each coupling. Even if the bladder contains little urine whilst intercourse takes place, excess penile length may cause bruising .

If the bladder hasn't been totally emptied before intercourse, urine might impede comfortable intercourse. The cervix will also become distressed.

A wide pelvis helps in child-bearing and easy birthing. If baby's head is larger than the exit route, Caesarean section may be better than a very long labour. It may pass through the cervical canal and vaginal canal all right, but the actual vaginal opening may be very badly stressed. Sometimes an episiotomy is performed cleanly slitting the vaginal opening backwards rather than let it tear and be more difficult to sew up neatly.

Every woman who has had an episiotomy knows it, and feels it to have left a much weaker perineum. Scars can harbour infection more readily and can often nick or split on intercourse. Plenty of lubricated foreplay over a few days should help prepare the vagina to resume full penile penetration. This must be gentle and the entire shaft of the penis lubricated as well as inside the vagina. If injury does occur and any bacteria are present on the perineal skin then a blood-borne infection can begin. Bottle Washing before and after foreplay and full intercourse limits bacteria and stops bacterial and non-bacterial cystitis.

Scars, whether natural or medical, heal slowly after birth because that area is seldom absolutely dry. Vaginal mucous, sweat, droplets of urine and fecal farting make the perineum quite a moist, bacterially laden area preventing fast recovery from childbirth.

An episiotomy can delay the resumption of intercourse after birth by three or four months and can also make the simple act of sitting down extremely uncomfortable. Women often suffer silently from its after-effects. Don't!

And it isn't only external scarring! Unseen injuries to the vagina and cervix may have healed badly. The cervix may have torn or not shrunk back so the penis bangs it and splits it again resulting in infection. If you feel that you have not recovered comfortable intercourse in the six months following childbirth, or there is cystitis, infection, soreness or pain inside, this must be reported. Get further opinions until someone does find a cause for the trouble. No matter how small the reason is - it's not the doctor's pain, go ahead and request repair to whatever has been found. Lifelong damage can be done in childbirth.

Childbirth has 'fashions'! Waterbirths for instance! In the 20th century most births were done lying down, now many young women have reverted to ancient traditions including standing up and minimal drugs. Whatever is agreed there may still be some perineal damage affecting sex for a long time. Take it easy and ensure excellent hygiene. Read up!

Conclusion

I must end such a section by begging the reader to take out private health insurance from an early adult age because so many sad ladies find their way to me for counselling in utter despair. The State health services are not always reliable and before gynaecological trouble sets in (if it does) that is the time to take out insurance. If you do it once you have become ill, that illness will not be acceptable to the health insurance company.

CHAPTER FOUR

4 Desires, Despairs and Diseases

How do you know if you desire intercourse? If you are a man your penis swells up and throbs, if you're a woman your vagina secretes a varying amount of sticky, clear lubricating mucous to assist penetration.

Babies are not wanted each time intercourse happens but sexual desire is equally intense and grows over the years of prime sexual activity. Female desire declines with age as hormone activity lessens and their mate becomes less attractive! Men remain fertile but can experience penile dysfunction. If you are lucky enough to be in a stimulating, responsive and healthy sexual liaison, then faithful intercourse becomes a very special bond.

If you are unlucky enough to have frequent sexually induced cystitis then you know frustration, desperation and discomfort. It can lead to a deep, deep well of unhappiness and sexual desire will certainly drop.

Forget any anal intercourse because bowels teem with billions of potentially lethal bacteria so whether a penis, sex toy or a finger is inserted there, it will come out absolutely coated with fecal deposit. Transfer this forward or into any other orifice and resulting infections will put her out of sexual activity for several weeks.

Sexual infections can arise at any time, even between faithful partners. Your own body, under all sorts of conditions favourable to bacteria, can start discharges, soreness, dryness and infection all by itself.

Sexual infections make you feel low and having to forgo sexual release is quite bad enough, but it also risks transmittance to your partner and may have already happened even before the first symptoms showed. Frequent bouts of yeast, cystitis, warts, herpes and discharges in general can really get you to screaming pitch and terrible despair.

No-one, but no-one, can fully appreciate life-long memories of wrecked holidays and outings on which, to all outward appearances, you and your partner are in seventh heaven when inwardly you are both enduring misery.

It is hateful to have to keep going back to the doctor when yet another bout starts. Each time you always think it's the last; each time you try so hard to get a positive attitude and put the past behind you; each time you're wrong and you search and search for the cure. A patient partner may snap and go off or maybe you put all care aside and fling yourself into his arms for lovemaking which is too fast for satisfaction, imperils the early effectiveness of the medication, is unhygienic, and only lengthens the problem.

Every discharge or reddened vulva may have a different bacterial source, so don't make the mistake of telling your doctor you've got 'X' again when it *may* now be 'Y' if it's put under a microscope. Never take it for granted that you have another attack of thrush: it could be a heavy hormonal discharge of vaginal epithelial cells instead.

You must get a vaginal examination and swabs. Use combinations of the doctor, the gynaecologist and the Genito-Urinary Clinic. Swabs should be pain-free - after all they're only long cotton buds - and taken from the cervix, the middle vagina and the vulva.

Trichomonas

This is a parasite living in moist areas. It can be transmitted from male to female and vice versa during intercourse, therefore behaving like a ping-pong ball. Once inside the vagina it lives within the mucous secretions, or even on the wall of the vagina. Men are usually symptom free but it can ping-pong.

Symptoms are vaginal flooding from brownish, frothy, itchy, smelly liquid. Without fast treatment it may worsen into cystitis and you won't quite know what to do with yourself with a combination of stinging, flooding and irritation!

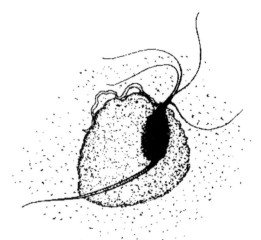

Trichomonas Vaginalis

For heaven's sake don't be tempted by intercourse at such a time! Go to a VD unit, special clinic or Genito-Urinary clinic where swabs will be taken and oral treatment with Flagyl dispensed. Trich will not abate with any other treatment.

When Trich, even without symptoms, is in the long male urethra, it can reach the prostate gland and just keep on being transmitted into a woman through ejaculation. Flagyl is necessary for both partners for at least a week. Trichomonal parasites die on contact with dry air so an on-site microscope is essential. Sometimes gonorrhoea links up with trichomonal parasites and if gonorrhoea remains undiscovered it invades the cervical canal, uterus and Fallopian tubes. Once embedded here, gonococcal infection will add high fever, nausea and pain to your discharge symptoms and inflame the wall of the tubes leading to infertility. Fast treatment with Penicillin is the remedy. Mercury preparations were used until antibiotics arrived but invariably the patient died from such poisonous treatment!

Something Completely Innocent

Bran fibre stimulates bowel action but bran molecules travel everywhere else in the bloodstream. It can overload urine agitating the bladder to eject it as an irritant. It can increase vaginal mucous and also cause stuffy noses! Diagnosis is impossible in a lab, check your dietary intake yourself and monitor changes. Too much brown bread and pure fibre may increase mucous. Interestingly, too much bran actually causes constipation when it clogs up intestines and slows fecal movement there. Beware too much so-called healthy living!

Many innocuous discharges can irritate the perineum and urethra causing cystitis or frequency.

Candida Albicans

Let's look at a fungus now. We all know it - vaginal thrush, of course, also known as Candida Albicans, yeast infection or Monilia.

Candida is a native of our whole body *all* the time. Blood-borne, it can be tested there and also from urine, vagina, ears, nose, throat, tongue, finger and toe-nails. It is competitive with bacteria in our gut but if the immune system is compromised for any reason like mercury teeth fillings, illness, stress, tiredness, loss of sleep, antibiotics, steroids, anaesthetics, diabetes, sugary/yeasty diet or practically anything else, Candida will surge over bacteria.

Vaginal Symptoms. Labia and vulva becomes dark purply-red, itchy and stiff. Hair follicles itch unmercifully but, don't scratch, or lichenized patches of labial skin may irritate for years and need constant steroid creams.

Stringy, creamy mucous itches like crazy and moves all over the perineum making things like episiotomy scars or hemorrhoids very sore. Equally, severe Thrush may have no discharge but just swelling. Anal irritation increases with smelly mucous.

Wash discharge off quickly every few hours with a bottle of cool or cold water poured down the perineum whilst you sit on the toilet. Dab it absolutely dry - really bone dry with discardable kitchen towel, **not** toilet paper because that will leave little bits behind. If you dry it with a cloth at this highly infective state the cloth will need to be changed each time so kitchen towel is probably the most sensible **just** for a day or so.

Don't walk anywhere!

Sit down and sit back. Wear a long, loose skirt and no underwear for maximum first aid and minimum spread of discharge.

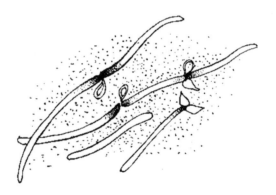

Candida / Yeast

Candida / Yeast

Thrush/yeast, microscopically looks like very fine spaghetti, tied or looped at intervals with thread. It is always wise to have a vaginal swab to confirm its presence because it is possible to have mild thrush without a readily seen discharge.

In terms of medical treatment, you will be given any one of a three to seven-day course of Gynodaktarin, Diflucan, Canesten or Nystatin pessaries or cream. Orally,

Nystatin tablets, Sporanox capsules, Diflucan, Itraconazole and Fluconazole are better because Systemic yeast infection requires systemic treatment. Certainly, if you need a course of antibiotics for something and are yeast-prone, you should take oral preventive measures alongside the antibiotics.

Patients are more aware of the part they themselves play in causing their own thrush and simple cool treatment and rest is very helpful at this stage of an upsurge.

Cervical Polyps

By the time you get your first diagnosed and treated cervical polyp you may well already know that you are inclined to be a 'polypy' person. Perhaps you had nasal polyps as a child or teenager. There are several sorts; large pendulous things growing singly, or groups of smaller ones looking like the surface of the moon.

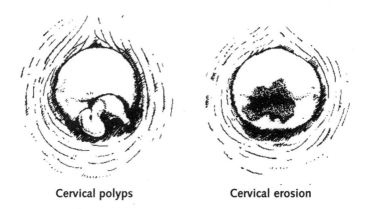

Cervical polyps   **Cervical erosion**

They can take ages to develop or arrive in a matter of weeks. When the discharge from them is sufficient to maintain a steady liquid drip, bacteria may thrive in it and urinary twinges or full-blooded cystitis will start.

Intercourse can puncture and split polyps and there may be unusual spots of blood on the sheets. This is another sure sign of any sort of vaginal or cervical growth and should never be ignored. It's there to be helpful

Go for a gynaecological examination. Depending upon its size a polyp can be twisted or frozen off, both simple, quick and pain free. Painkillers will ease any aching. Polyps are always sent for analysis.

Afterwards, sloughing of the cervix, much like the end of a period, eases as the raw patch heals. Resting helps a lot to dry it up so sit or lie with legs apart. If the polyp had harboured infection, then a course of appropriate antibiotics would be indicated.

Cervical Erosion

The cervical canal leading to the uterus can have an overgrowth of cells. If cystitis, discomfort, soreness accompany it, then the erosion should be cautherised to its base. This can mean two or three trips at intervals for treatment.

If it is large enough to impede menstrual flow then you should ask for a general anaesthetic in a Day Care Unit.

Doctors are lazy about removing erosion, arguing that it's a common thing and best left alone. This is quite unacceptable when intercourse hurts or soreness, discharge and cystitis are factors. Be firm about removal.

Search until someone agrees to your request. Here's a real case for private health insurance.

Recovery is as for polyps. There may be considerable sloughing and you should certainly rest for a week, especially if you have had a general anaesthetic. Don't attempt intercourse until after the next menstrual bleed. More sloughing may come away with that. Do remember to go back six weeks later for a clearance check because repeat treatment may be needed.

Wart Virus

This is very common. If you are sexually active you should regard everything on your hands with suspicion, warts included. A young nurse recently put on the children's ward contracted a couple of finger warts.

Out of the blue came a nasty vaginal discharge, pain and cystitis. Raging at her boyfriend, accusing him of 'giving' something to her she marched off to the hospital gynaecologist who found a nest of warts on the cervix exuding a runny liquid laden with virus. Warts can locate anywhere on the perineum or in any orifice including bowels.

In lovemaking, finger warts caught from children could have transmitted the virus during later intercourse. Warts were frozen off her cervix and fingers but if the virus has penetrated the epithelial cervical or vaginal lining then she may expect further bouts until it wanes of its own accord. Incubation for the wart virus

Condyloma Acuminatum can vary from one to six months. That this nurse was well until a month after developing her finger warts on the children's ward shows how virulent warts are. Household pets get warts, too. Ask the vet to treat them immediately and be extra vigilant for the human householders! Lifestyle is vital for correct diagnosis!

Herpes

Once it colonises it will remain for years, each attack less distressing and acutely painful than before but it is highly contagious and intercourse should only happen with barrier contraception like condoms. *Lysine*, available in all pharmacies acts as both treatment and daily prevention. Take a heavy dose for treatment and much less as prevention once Herpes is diagnosed. Whoever gave it to you needs investigating or if previously diagnosed, you could talk to a lawyer.

Carcinoma of the Cervix

Cancer of the cervix can start early, even fifteen, if intercourse begins early. The younger you commence intercourse, the greater your chances of cervical removal for cancer and decreased fertility. Having frequent intercourse with uncircumcised men also increases chances of cell changes and cervical cancer. Cervical cancer is almost unknown in societies like the Jews where male circumcision is practised.

Give your body chemistry a chance to grow up fully so that it can repel malignant cells. Get on with sports, hobbies, academic work and travel until you are twenty when cervical strength peaks. Once you start intercourse you will want more sex, so try hard not to start early. I think that co-educational schools have placed upon girls unfair and dangerous sexual pressures. Classwork suffers and so can health.

Cancerous cells of several kinds can grow in the cervical canal or very visibly on the vaginal side of the cervix. You may not know that you have a problem because in its early stages cervical cancer can be symptom free, but as it grows there will be all sorts of symptoms including urinary infection, cystitis, back ache, discharge, bleeding between periods or after intercourse, pain on intercourse and period-type aches.

Such symptoms will worsen if a gynaecologist doesn't 'find' you in good time. The cancer will spread to include uterus, ovaries, and then onward round the body.

At best you may lose your cervix and fertility; at worst you may die. Take sexual health care and behaviour very seriously. Being regretful in your 30's and 40's is far too late!

Pelvic Infections and the IUD

Almost any heavy bacterial infection of the vagina can rise up through the cervical canal into the uterus and Fallopian tubes; leaking bacteria from ovarian cysts can travel down the tubes into the uterus.

Bacterial clumps which embed themselves in uterine walls spread infection to pelvic organs. Infection in Fallopian tubes is called Salpingitis.

If you know that you are prone to vaginal infections and discharges, it is crazy to have any kind of intra-uterine device fitted for contraception. Bacteria are not stupid, they will choose the fastest route and the string hanging off IUDs will help them spread quickly.

An IUD prevents conception by keeping the cervical canal slightly dilated preventing a fertilized egg from embedding itself in the uterine wall. If cystitis or discharge or any pain begins with the insertion of an IUD, don't hesitate - have it out straight away.

Those women already scarred both externally and internally by birthing and medical injuries should not contemplate the IUD. Old birth scars welcome marching germs! An IUD may open up an old scar, chafe, or just be an additional hazard. The string harbours rising bacteria and cystitis or discharges may start.

Discharges from pelvic infections encourage Neisseria gonorrhoea, Chlamydia trachomatis and anaerobic bacteroides or cocci. Bowel bacteria like E. Coli or streptococcus can also cause pelvic infections and are mainly self caused by ineffective hygiene. Tap water in third world countries can carry bacteria and parasites so filter, boil and store this water ready for Bottle Washing if you live in such surroundings.

Pelvic infections require improved hygiene and plenty of antibiotics, so take plenty of Nystatin oral tablets if you're thrush prone, plenty of fluids, plenty of mineral and vitamin supplements, plenty of effective hygiene and plenty of rest. All bacteria spread faster if you walk round - don't. Sit or lie down during the treatments and don't have intercourse. You'll feel too ill anyway!

Normal Discharges

Personal vaginal secretions vary according to the time of the month, whether on the Pill, pregnant, having intercourse regularly or sporadically.

The older you become, the drier your vagina. If you have recently had a discharge, the vaginal epithelium may not have recovered its natural flow and the pH balance may still be upset, so attempts at intercourse will need a good lubricating jelly and some care.

The discharge that most sexually active women have is a thick white mucous. It varies in amount, but can be heavy and sticky. This discharge is Non Infective Leucorrhoea and increases during pregnancy. It can be contained by a full Bottle Wash and vaginal clean morning and evening. Don't EVER use a bidet.

Ask for swabs if you are worried, but if hygiene is good the chances of negative bacterial results are also good. Whether you have a very heavy discharge, a dry, burning vagina or variations in between, you must investigate. Discharges and vaginal conditions are so quick to influence the bladder that examination and appropriate treatment can quickly become necessary.

Examination

The most comfortable position for vaginal examination is called Dorsal. It is unpleasant to go straight into a left lateral (side) and expose the anal opening. The speculum, which is used to prop open the vaginal walls, should be warm and inserted first, if possible, before fingers, so as not to re-arrange the mucous needed for cytological smears. Help by keeping your arms at your side - the instinct is to put them behind your head - and taking good, if forced, breath to try to relax the abdominal muscles. If they are very tense, and the vagina too, it will be difficult to examine you thoroughly.

Of course, if you visit regularly, then examination is less of a tense affair. I am astounded at the numbers of women who haven't been examined in three or more years, yet some silly doctor has been packing them with antibiotics or has missed some vital gynaecological symptom like back ache and failed to refer to an expert. It can be helpful to have access to several medical personnel. I use private health insurance, two general practitioners, one National Health and one private, two gynaecologists, and access to the special clinic in a teaching hospital. I rarely see any of them, but in past years of suffering, such access helped enormously to deal correctly and swiftly with my highly-sensitive skin, bad childbirth and cystitis.

If you have a vagina you must use gynaecologists or the G.U. Clinic. A sexually active vagina needs more attention, not less.

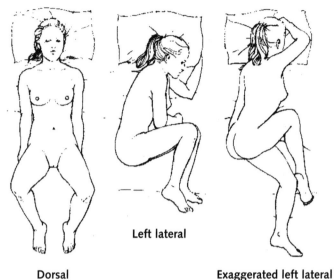

Left lateral

Dorsal **Exaggerated left lateral**

Gynaecological examination

Bacteria and Their Origins

There are many unusual bacteria that can find their way up the vagina to the cervix. The VD or special clinic may not check for unusual bacteria but always talk during the examination asking about red areas, erosions, polyps etc.

Here are common bacteria and their origin.

Klebsiella A group with several strains but most usually waterborne as external contamination, or from swallowing bad water.

Pseudomonas Aeruginosa (frequently found in hospital departments)

Neisseria Pharyngis, Catarrhalis (both possible from oral sex), Gonorrhoea.

Proteus Mirabilis, Vulgaris (enjoy an alkaline medium. Also found in renal pelvic condition and septicaemia).

Streptococci Fecalis (from bowels), Haemolytic (from skin infections), Pyogenes (from nose and throat), Pneumoniae (from lungs).

E.Coli (Escherichia coliform) Fecal serotypes are 01, 02, 04, 06, 07, 025, 050 (from the small intestines and bowels).

Staphylococcus Aureus (found in the lower respiratory tract), Epidermitis, Saprophyheus, Albus (from bladder catheterization).

Yeasts (Candida/monilia) Albicans, Stellatoidea, Tropicalis, Krusei, Pseudo Tropicalis, Parapsilosis, Guilliermondii, Norvegensis.

Rhodoturula Rubra.

Trichomonas Vaginalis Mycoplasma Hominis, Toralopsis Glabrata, Castellii, Inconspicua, Hominii, Saccharomyces Cervisae. Genitalium, Urilyticum.

Haemophilus Inluenzae Parainfluenzae, Vaginalis, Ducreyi (soft chancroid).

Chlamydia Trachomatis Chlamydia B. (a type frequently found in birds and can be passed to people in contact with domestic/wild birds).

Gardnerella Vaginalis Otherwise known as Corynebacterium Vaginale or H. Vaginalis (thin discharge)

Mycoplasmas (see IC book)

Bacterial vaginosis (from overheated perineums)

In 1966 Gordan et. Al. showed the frequency of occurrence of various organisms in normal vaginal flora, taken from a sample of women.

Haemophilus Vaginalis	9.8
Corynebacterium (diptheroids)	39.0
Mycoplasma (PPLO)	15.3
Lactobacilli (Doderlein)	81.0
Coliform	12.2
Aerobic Streptococci	24.2
Strep Fecalis	0.0
Anaerobic organisms	21.0
Staph Aureus	0.0
Candida	9.7

All organisms on the chart can overgrow and cause discharges with or without urinary involvement.

Daily Rules Preventing Infections

Any diseases or discharges can cause cystitis. Prevention of such disasters, discomfort and disease is miles better than agonies of mind and body when yet another attack looks imminent.

Why not take simple daily care of the vagina and perineum just as you would your teeth, face and hair?

'Because of its proximity to the genital organs, the bladder is often involved in gynaecological disorders.' OR 'Gynaecological disorders are often associated with bladder disorders.' wrote Sir John Peel and Professor Brudenell in 1961!

Is this understood in today's medical schools? Are common sense and logic used in diagnosis? Maybe not.

There is no doubt that my early and subsequent work on cystitis and associated conditions has broken new ground not only for sufferers but also for many specialists. Common sense and simple preventative directives help everyone.

So here to prevent the diseases we have just looked at are some useful tips.

Some Prevention

Trichomonas
1. Toilet water contains Trichomonas. Place a sheet of toilet paper in the pan to stop fecal backsplash if the pan is deep, before passing a stool.
2. If the pan is unusually shallow and you need to flush at an intermediate stage, get up and wait for the flushing water to subside. Don't flush parasites all over the vulva!

Full Bottle Washing Procedure -
always done before any sex!

1. Use toilet paper straight not scrunched up.
2. Stand up at the basin. Wash and scrub your hands with soap and hot water.
3. Re-soap **one** hand lathering the anal orifice only, nowhere else, from behind. Use only a pure soap, not perfumed, coloured, antiseptic or deodorized. The safest is either a glycerine or a white unperfumed baby soap.
4. Rinse that hand very well under **running** warm water. Don't use the plug!
5. Fill a 500ml mineral water bottle with very warm, not hot, water. NOT a milk bottle, carton, larger bottle, watering can, jug or glass! Water must be very warm because fecal material from the bowels is greasy and won't wash off with cool water. If you are out of your own bathroom and you forgot to take your bottle, acquire one from the bar, the very, very last resort is the bathroom mug. Wash it out well and use several fill-ups to do the same job as the bottle, which is:
6. Return to and sit on the toilet, relaxing your back bone in a **pelvic tilt** as the lowest part of your bottom, downwards. Pour the warm water **from the front** down the labia, vulva and perineum and with the spare hand clean around the inner labia finally ensuring that **all** the soap is off the anus. Don't lean backwards.
7. Pat all dry with a wash-cloth, not toilet paper as it leaves bits behind to gather

daily anal mucous.

8. If the vagina needs cleaning out, fill up the bottle again but with lukewarm water and hook out as much mucous as you can with the third finger. Pat thoroughly dry again. Never just do a vaginal clean without a full wash EXCEPT after sex, because germs will get pushed into the vagina.

Bottle Washing should be done twice a day and always before ANY intercourse whenever or wherever it happens.

Bacteria from the bowels constantly leak out in mucous or wind and pre-sex Bottle Washing should be done just before intercourse starts, even its 4.00am after a disco.

Candida Albicans
(also called thrush, monilia or yeast)

Control upsurges by:

1. Having mercury amalgam teeth fillings safely removed by a knowledgeable anti-mercury dentist to boost the immune system.
2. Removing glucose and sugar from your diet because candida lives on it.
3. Removing as much man-refined carbohydrate food from your diet as possible because it converts to sugar in the body. Flour, pasta and rice should be decreased.
4. Checking if the Pill can be linked. There is no doubt in practice that Pill-users are a big group of thrush sufferers, so if thrush starts and arises frequently whilst you are on the Pill you must contemplate coming off it.
5. Taking Nystatin oral tablets or Fluconazole capsules every time you need a course of antibiotics, as a preventative.
6. Vaginal acid/alkaline balance is also important. Thrush grows in an alkaline environment, blood is alkaline - so is the vagina around a period. Introduce a lactic acid pessary or a good natural yoghurt or a therapeutic acid-based vaginal gel high up to the cervix at night before and after a period to maintain acidity.

All of the following points help prevent Candida /Yeast

- Eat three or four tablespoons of live yoghurt twenty minutes before any meal to line the stomach with lactobacilli.
- Don't eat sweets or chocolates.

- Don't drink alcohol, canned sodas or juices. Alcohol converts to sugar.
- Avoid cheeses and other yeast/fermenting foods.
- Shower, don't soak in a hot bath.
- Swimming in treated water has an antiseptic action on the perineal skin and inside the vagina. It will promote the growth of yeast.
- Wearing lycra/nylon clothing such as leotards for keep fit, jogging, dancing and so on heightens body heat and sweating. Thrush loves a hot body.
- Sunbathing in a lycra/nylon suit promotes thrush .
- Sexual intercourse can ping-pong thrush. It is sexually transmittable. Skin friction in intercourse raises vaginal and body temperature. Cool the vagina after sex with a bottle of cold water.
- Jeans cause perineal perspiration. Jean seams add clitoral and urethral bruising. Throw them away.
- Any restrictive outer clothing like trousers or tailored skirts prevents cooling air from drying the vulva. Wear looser clothing.
- Tights and nylon panties also cause sweating and stop air. Only wear stockings, suspender belts and cotton panties.
- Go without underwear whenever possible. Slips or petticoats are fine.
- Don't sit all day on the edge of the office chair. Allow the vulva to breathe and dry out.
- Cut pubic hair to half an inch every four or five weeks at the same time as you do toenails, because pubic hair retains perineal sweat and the enlarged hair follicles trap fungus.
- Bedding should be warm but 'breathing'. Use cotton sheets and blankets if you share a double bed. Terylene duvets will increase sweating though down duvets may be all right.
- Wear cotton nighties - not pyjamas and certainly no undies in bed.

Having said all that, large numbers of women have 'deeper' thrush, thrush that sits in the gut in a permanent overload' situation. Antibiotics, diabetes, mercury fillings, steroids, anaesthetics, stress, tiredness, sleep deprivation, death illnesses and yeast allergy are some deep background causes of ongoing Candida.

Safe removal of mercury fillings, less hormonal activity, anti-yeast allergy injections and sensible rotating diet all keep me quite free of it now.

That we have this combination of self-help and medical help for thrush is due to an immense increase in thrush over the past twenty-five years. Modern life is entirely responsible and information must be relayed to sufferers and doctors. Thrush is preventable.

Wart Virus and Herpes

As with all sexually transmittable diseases, you should be absolutely honest before having intercourse with a stranger about the presence of a discharge, or warts, herpes, chlamydia, thrush, syphilis, gonorrhoea, pubic lice (crabs), worms, Aids, and scabies.

The sheath is the only barrier able to protect sexual organs. Herpes upsurges should make you forgo sex for the three or four-week period of its presence. Take Lysine tablets as daily prevention and more in an attack.

Anyone with a lip sore should be avoided like the plague. No kissing, no touching and put restrictions on towels, napkins, crockery, cutlery, with those items being separately washed away from others in the home. Sadly, the Communion cup now becomes suspicious and intinction /dipping chalices stop transference of disease.

Warts on the hands or any hand contact with warty genitalia are contagious. Hot water, antiseptic, antiseptic soap and a scrubbing brush should be employed on the hands at the first opportunity and thereafter. Go for a vaginal and cervical swab to check out possible transference of the hand infection internally. Warts internally and externally can and should be cauterized or frozen. If you work with, or have children who grow a wart, treatment must be sought in case someone sexually active has skin contact with them.

Cervical Erosion

As I said previously, this will drip and its only treatment is to seek medical help. However, if you know how to clean out the vagina you can restrain and restrict the drip a little bit and be more comfortable.

Use the full Bottle-Washing method scrupulously to remove invasive bowel-perineal bacteria regularly. The cool water vaginal bottle wash will help limit the drip. Put an eggcup full of Betadine liquid, an iodine-based medication available from most pharmacies, into the Bottle Wash which will limit bacterial growth maintaining comfort until surgical removal.

Pelvic Infections

Again hygiene, as per the bottle washing, will prevent all rising infections from the perineum. This is the commonest route for such infections so take the daily bottle washing with great seriousness - it is protecting all the pelvic organs both renal and productive.

Normal Discharges

There is volume and colour variation throughout the monthly cycle, but if at any time this non-bacterial discharge (do get it checked if it is too heavy) causes slight irritation, uncomfortable wetness or soreness then wash it out just as previously discussed. You will be bottle washing after a bowel movement anyway, so follow it with a vaginal bottle wash, but a freshener at night-time is nice and, as you'll see later, is incorporated into pre- and post-intercourse routines.

If Sir John Peel, the Queen's past gynaecologist and myself are both in favour of absolutely 'scrupulous hygiene', you can bet it's the right thing to do! So please work away at the proper perineal hygiene taught here, it takes 15-20 seconds. Don't ever use a bidet, don't squat in the bath, don't sit over the sink or any other manner of procedure!! You must do the bottle washing absolutely precisely as I have described not what you think you can improve upon!

E.Coli Cystitis

All adult women, and also children with bacteria in their urine samples, should do a full Bottle Wash precisely as described. It will prevent cystitis. I am not in favour of drinking Cranberry juice and making rich companies even richer. It is not effective, can cause bladder thrush from the sugars and is no substitute for washing off germs as surgeons do before they operate!

However, if you find Cranberry tablets helpful in your particular circumstances perhaps because you are confined to a wheelchair then go ahead and try.

E. Coli multiplies by itself every 12 minutes continuously and can colonise anywhere warm and moist like the perineum. Cystitis after intercourse caused by fecal coliforms can start from twelve to fifty five hours later if washing before sex has been non-existent or stupidly lax. Infection is more likely to occur in women whose perineums are shorter between the vulva and anus allowing quicker, easier baterial travel.

Only Bottle Washing stops this travel and urinary infections. Its cheap, quick and works anywhere with a toilet and basin.

Bottle Washing will revolutionise your existence!

CHAPTER FIVE

5 Contraceptives

Women inevitably organise their own contraception. Even so, mistakes will always be made, but abortion and the Morning-after Pill can erase newly fertilised eggs preventing embryo formation. If you don't want a child, don't hesitate to make use of these modern advances if you have made a mistake and don't worry over scare stories telling you of lifelong psychological damage! It's not true. If you don't want a baby for all your own reasons, then you will not be upset at a heavier period that month.

Abortions after twelve weeks are certainly more traumatic both medically and mentally so seek earlier treatment and be sure. After twelve weeks my advice is to go through with the pregnancy but put the baby to a desperate, infertile couple if possible and get on with whatever life course you are on. It's hard but realistic. Be certain that rearing a child under impossible circumstances doesn't do you or it any good at all.

Contraceptive choice is varied. The Pill, condoms/sheath, Coil, Diaphragm/Cap, hormone implants, hormone patches, cervical sponges, foams/gels, ovulation control, old herbal remedies and of course, the old withdrawal method and cold water douche have all had their place in female contraceptive history. There are good books to read on the subject. In later life both men and women have surgical choices of sterilisation such as tubal ligation and vasectomy. Two or three years after menopause, contraception comes naturally with thinning uterine lining and decreased provision of eggs for fertilisation. This doesn't mean an end to intercourse. Hormone Replacement Therapy and lubricant gels enable enriched sexual activity still requiring all the hygiene rules. Bacteria take no account of human age: cystitis can still start.

Historically, drug companies, spurred by thoughts of profit, new medical knowledge and engineering processes, have continuously devised and tested methods of contraception. Spermicidal creams, foams and pessaries were marketed as non-prescribable so that effective contraception was instantly available. Condoms for men have always been non-prescribable and widely available.

The coil was marketed in the late 1960s as a new foolproof method for those unable to tolerate the Pill. It had the major disadvantage of needing skilled medical insertion. Heavy monthly bleeding nasty infections and occasional coil dispersal out of the uterus were also drawbacks.

'Morning after' injections of heavy doses of hormones and the new cervical sponges with spermicidal agents are more recent additions to the market.

Not all contraceptives suit every patient. If I were to map out the contraceptive requirements and practices of any female in an idealistic way it would be:

1. Abstinence until nineteen to twenty-one years old to lessen risks of cervical illnesses and cancer.
2. The sheath until a strong regular relationship develops.
3. Six months of any year on a low dose Pill and six months of sheath and sponge combinations.
4. Find a suitable, well-tolerated Pill.
5. Perhaps an experimental time with the coil after careful discussion with a good gynaecologist and all relevant individual health assessments made. But preferably not.
6. The vaginal sponge, sheath, mini Pill.
7. Careful cool water washing out of the vagina in older age.

There is no hard and fast way of recommending contraception. It has to be individual choice knowing what suits you best. From my engagement, the sheath was an occasional protection, but mostly withdrawal. There was no cystitis or discomfort of any sort, which I now put down to wanting to smell nice before sex for my fiancé, passing urine afterwards because I would be travelling and then showering or bathing to cover up my activities before facing the world! My vagina also had plenty of time to recover - weeks!

From the marriage night on, though, I didn't have to leave my new husband's side so, without having been told the health importance of cleaning up, I didn't. Additionally, my doctor had suggested the vaginal foam Emko as a contraceptive since I had had major abdominal surgery in my early twenties. I used Emko for three years without ever thinking to link it with cystitis or vaginal stinging. We were entirely at the mercy of doctors in those days, there was no literature whatsoever or any media coverage of intimate problems.

Emko was one of several spermicidal foams using mercury as the spermicide. Mercury is known to kill or maim sperm hence its contraceptive value. Vapour from teeth fillings settles in Testes damaging sperm and contributing to male infertility because sperm head-bang instead of making a straight entry into the egg.

With nasty, frequent bouts of cystitis, lovemaking in between and no known cause as yet for this dreadful suffering, I was frantic to make up for the two or three weeks lost every four weeks to cystitis attacks. Passionate sexual make-up sessions would have left a swollen, raw and still small vagina very open to chemical contamination with additional inflammation from the foam contraceptive and sexual thrusting. There were seven years of doctors, hospitals, operations, antibiotics, pain, crying, frustration, screams and dreadful fear of the next attack starting.

A three-week spell on a high estrogen Pill added a stone in weight leaving me dizzy and tearful. My body took six months to recover from it so I steered clear of the Pill for years. There were no mini-pills then.

With constant cystitis and thrush my opera career faded and it was decided to start a family whilst I was so confined to the house. Contraception became unnecessary and the immediate pregnancy blessedly brought nine cystitis-free months. We know now that extra hormonal padding prevented easy bacterial travel and improved immune responses. It ended with an unnecessary Caesarean section by a greedy obstetrician and a long convalescence.

Withdrawal, Emko and the sheath were used when required but by now antibiotics for cystitis were causing permanent thrush. Sex was more off the marital menu than on.

When mini-Pills were invented I had a couple of sessions of Minovlar before and after the birth of my son with some better success than the earlier brush with the higher dose Pill. But then my husband went abroad to work and this began eight years of partings and irregular sex between us, so I had no need of daily contraception.

Apart from wishing time and again for a less sensitive metabolism, I have come off lightly in terms of any permanent reaction or damage from man-made contraceptives. Emko has not caused permanent medical damage but it's effects and atrocious sexual hygiene helped ruin our marital bonding.

Saying to my then husband that I'd had more than enough female trouble and operations for one woman, I wanted him to take over permanent contraceptive responsibility. So one Christmas, I bought him a vasectomy and ended my own contraceptive headaches for the duration of the marriage.

However, my marriage broke up, so this was not to be the end of my contraceptive responsibility. So for a while I settled on a non-prescribable vaginal tablet, reasonably priced. As a well-taught consumer I obeyed the packet's instructions and inserted a tablet high up to the cervix before penetration but on several occasions it caused soreness and urinary reactions after intercourse. By now my knowledge of cystitis had improved from research and writing on it and I was plainly reacting to the chemicals in the tablets, just as I obviously had with the Emko years earlier but was then unaware of the mercury spermicidal link.

Contraception has ceased since the menopause and I use cool water Bottle Washing within minutes of intercourse ending. Sperm is killed anyway in cool or cold water. Perhaps I had not been truly fertile since my inverted uterus, I'd love to know, but there is no fertility measurement test.

With much personal sadness, I should add that I have been as careful and hygienic as possible, once I knew how vital it is! But I wish that life itself had been kinder. I expect men to pay attention to hygiene and kindly responsibilities to their female partner, women respond to being cherished. More women divorce men than vice versa because we simply will not tolerate bad behaviour these days. Both sexes should respect each other and take joint sexual health responsibilities seriously.

Travel, choice, unclean blood products, homosexual and bisexual intercourse encourage HIV Aids. Saying NO sometimes just might stave off a pregnancy and a dangerous one night stand. Bottle Washing / male showering will wash off fecal and foreskin germs.

Desires and Diseases are individually variable. I have met countless women in my adult social life and, of course, in my work with cystitis. There are women who start the Pill in their teens and have happily stayed on it all their sexual lives. Many healthy women have needlessly come off the Pill in a scare only to find a reaction to the replacement contraceptive or even an unwanted pregnancy.

All of us have met someone with a drug reaction. The key to successful Pill-taking is a really good gynaecologist who will stick with you as you search for the most suitable brand.

Rest periods are important for regular Pill takers, six months off in every three years is a common recommendation. Coming off in order to get pregnant successfully requires three-month's use of an alternative contraceptive to give the uterus time to build up its nutritious lining. If the lining is too thin, a growing embryo cannot be nourished and it will abort itself.

Both partners should have mercury amalgam teeth fillings removed SAFELY by an anti-mercury dentist during this preparatory time. Conception is helped by placing a pillow under the buttocks after intercourse and resting like that for fifteen to twenty minutes. Every month for the first three months of pregnancy rest up or even go to bed because miscarriage is more likely to occur at the time your periods would have begun.

The coil / IUD needs medical insertion and removal which means delays. It can get lost and the string encourages vaginal infections. Nasty pelvic inflammatory diseases and cystitis can be traced to insertion of a coil, and if the doctor inserting it accidentally bends any part of the structure, then the uterus can be damaged.

It always strikes me as odd that men don't like rolling on a sheath yet how would they enjoy putting their legs in stirrups for a coil insertion and then wait for it to settle down in their system with, for instance, heavy bleeding or back ache? Or how would they enjoy anticipating when intercourse might occur and inserting a large rubber dome smothered with gel in good time? Furthermore, after sex, pull the whole mucky mess back down again, wash it off and put it away in a box until next time? Yuck!

No man I can think of would put up with all that and have the grace to be a good lover! Caps can harbour fecal residue from poor washing or absence of perineal hygiene before sex begins.

Perhaps some older men are better lovers than younger men because withdrawal of the penis just before ejaculation made for a bit more planning, design and control with more time to serve and please. So did calculating the point at which the sheath should be put on. Both ways encouraged lengthier and cleverer sexual prowess to forestall climax but were not foolproof against pregnancy.

However, once the Pill emerged as an unseen and effective contraceptive, young men had no such pressures and may have begun to lose sexual skills as a result. Skilled lovemaking lessens urethral and vaginal soreness.

All contraceptives are capable of causing urethritis and cystitis; all contraceptives are capable of causing various vaginal, cervical and uterine disorders. All contraceptives therefore, should be thoughtfully used by everyone.

Anytime that you have intercourse and can, with the help of this book, relate cystitis to that intercourse, it could be worthwhile checking out your contraceptive practice amongst other possible causes.

CHAPTER SIX

6 Recap

So you're about to have intercourse and you have made many thoughtful background preparations:

- A healthy set of reproductive organs
- A healthy set of renal organs
- A disease-free body
- An emptied bowel and bladder
- Clean teeth - (its nicer!)
- A tube of lubricating gel near by
- An aroused man!
- A cleaned perineum and properly bottle-washed anus
- A well lubricated vagina
- A well washed penis!
- An appropriate contraceptive
- Clean and smooth fingernails (him too!)
- Not too much acid alcohol circulating in the bloodstream!

PART TWO

Having Intercourse

CHAPTER SEVEN

7 Foreplay and Forethought

I am concerned that people have cystitis-free intercourse and a happy sex life, quite contrary to my own unwittingly self-caused sadnesses.

My mother only ever had one dose of mild cystitis in later life and I have no idea whether she ever washed before and after intercourse. Sexual intercourse was never discussed neither did I have sisters or brothers with whom to chat, and magazines, books and media items on cystitis were non-existent.

Today, things are much different and although cystitis is miserable, women no longer die from it nor is a lifetime of suffering necessary.

Attraction

Men and women prefer intercourse with someone who is nice to them: someone kind, clean and attractive to them.

Women don't know whether any man will be a good sexual partner until intercourse has happened a few times. And, of course, he himself is quite unaware whether his sexual ratings are excellent, average or poor because he doesn't have lessons from other males in making love. Reading porn and watching blue movies all night doesn't translate into personal rhythm or skill, this is either instinctive or acquired. Women are cheerful and encouraging in the main during lovemaking with a chosen partner. If he's not that brilliant, so what? He might improve! At least you are having intercourse and enjoying some parts of it. It takes a very extrovert and brave woman to change and improve a man's lovemaking, or even to tell him he's no good at all!

Of course, its not all one way, women need sexual skills too. A few other lovers would improve responses and teach different positions.

Prostitutes are in regular practice. They have to please because they are being paid to do so. A poorly performing customer matters not a jot if he doesn't know what to do with his hands or if he's got bad cigarette breath, or even if his penis is on the small side and doesn't reach high enough inside her.

Turn-offs

Such masculine inadequacies matter hugely in a regular sexual partnership. Fat stomachs, hairy noses, spitting, dirty hands, long dirty nails, smelly breath, a smelly penis, no small-talk or too much, and a poor idea of rhythm and timing are death to good regular sex. Conversely, face creams, hair nets, cucumbers on the eyes, nagging and a smelly vagina will likewise keep your man from your bed!

Regular practice, love and sexual health maintain bonding, pleasure and a lastingly loving relationship. If you are starting out on your sex life and reading this, I recommend buying a good honest sex manual with pictures, no porn videos or magazines.

Oral Sex

This is dealt with in Interstitial Cystitis, the third book. It is fraught with possible bacterial transference.

Fingerwork/Foreplay

Handwork or foreplay will relax and enlarge the vagina, but a young male 'broom handle' needs little encouragement. Do to each other anything that you both enjoy, except touching or penetrating the anus. It is perfectly possible to spend hours caressing, stroking, massaging any part of each other's body, particularly inside the vagina and around the penis.

Only a clean, scrubbed and well-rinsed hand should go near sensitive genitalia. If your partner usually likes some handwork, don't put hand cream on before you work on him, it may contain some chemical that could cause a mutual allergic reaction. Clean hands and lots of lubricant gel help an easier penetration. If non-bacterial cystitis is playing a part in association with sex, have a think about where hands are for most or part of the day. Is the coal dust really washed off or the photographic developer, paint, sand or garden spray? Chemicals from bathroom products build up and did the pre-sex shower occur?

The whole object of foreplay is to loosen up the vagina, attain easy penile penetration whilst reducing the possibility of vaginal bruising and non-bacterial sexual cystitis.

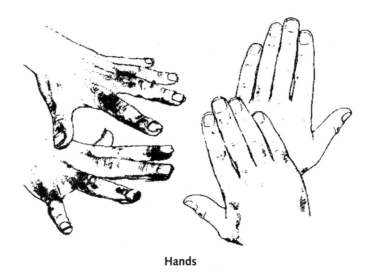

Hands

Penile Curvature

Very approximately, an erect male penis curves upwards, but if you were to stand ten naked erect men in a row and study penile curve there would be differences. Some won't curve at all but point away at a right angle; others will have a left or right curve and naturally the lengths and widths will be different. Others will curve slightly inwards.

Vaginal curving almost corresponds to penile curvature, but with a younger couple - he'll be at his most rigid and she'll be at her tightest - there's not a lot of room for easy movement. Vaginal elasticity is potentially great, but before childbirth, muscles are tighter and unyielding which means that, rather than absorb the impact, they can be bruised. If a penis doesn't roughly conform to your internal shape, thrusting may not cleanly use the gap between the vaginal walls so changing sexual positions helps avoid bruising one specific spot. Changing positions can simply involve shifting a bit more weight to one side by an inch or so, gymnastics are unnecessary!

Thin skin bruises more easily and so a vagina with thin layers may not protect the urethra adequately during intercourse. Bruised urethral nerve endings may bring on symptoms of urethritis and cystitis but without bacteria. Eating more, exercising less to encourage an extra six to ten pounds in weight may be an enormous help, if not the whole answer for many young women.

Penetration

If you are young and not so skilled at sex, it is important to find somewhere quiet, warm, and organise a time when you can relax totally.

Always make sure you have nearby a box of tissues, a tube of lubricating gel, a bath towel, an empty 500ml mineral water bottle for washing the perineum, a wash-cloth to dry with, and check out the condom situation. Don't put the telly on; it's the greatest sex killer of all time! Put a nice supper together - the snacky sort, not heavy! Throw a CD in the music centre, stick a candle in the holder and relax. (I once had a session to remember forever, thanks to the trombones and kettledrums of the Women's Royal Army Corps band playing on a summer's afternoon on the bandstand below the hotel!)

Use all unusual circumstances - life's happiest memories can be made of such and they really don't happen that often. If your boyfriend is more than casual and you have settled into a good steady affair, being as sure as you can be that he's not having it off with anyone else, try the vaginal sponge or go on the Pill. That way you will both take a fair share of the responsibility.

If you are not completely relaxed you may not always be well lubricated. Perhaps you've had a tiring day, or you weren't well last night and didn't sleep properly. Such things can affect vaginal secretion and erection, too. It's perfectly normal, but if your boyfriend's broom handle is to slide in and out easily and not bruise you, some lubricant gel will come in handy. Unfortunately, there is no jelly to help a flagging erection! Herbal Viagra-type products from health shops might if there is a regular flop!

Tell him if it hurts anywhere but otherwise aim at gently massaging the vulva, clitoris and vagina with the lubricant. There's nothing like vaginal wetness to drive a man crazy with delight and if you've started out a bit on the dry side, lubrication will relax your mind away from all fear of bruising and soreness. Vaginal secretions will respond and before you know it, five minutes have passed and you'll be reaching for the bath towel. Double it up and make sure it is well placed underneath, especially towards the backbone because liquids run along the seam of the perineum and gravity drops it off well past all the openings leaving an embarrassing stain or puddle somewhere.

Learning Skills

Before full penetration learn more about sexual preferences. One person tries something, the other reacts. One reaction brings more action and a wonderful 'body conversation ' begins. Young lovers are usually both inexperienced and underskilled. The 'wanting' of each other, the urgency to penetrate, brings only a brief physical satisfaction of minutes. There's much extra satisfaction to be had from foreplay, interplay and orchestration. Confidence will build as does the need for more sex when hormone levels increase with regular intercourse. If you've got plenty of time, use outside influences like music, candles, a lacy half-slip, perfume, (if you're not allergic to it, and likely to sneeze), suspenders, a pretty necklace, change the place you generally have sex; lie down, sit down, stand up, bend over, tell stories (not fibs), recount a special sexual moment. Enjoy your body conversations.

Health Warnings!

Some warnings: mouths and throats are not always well. Don't kiss if you have a cold sore, or if either has a sore throat, cold, oral thrush or any kind of sinusitis, tonsillitis or mouth infection. It really isn't fair to pass it on. HIV Aids can be blood-borne and genitally contracted. Make absolutely certain of the trustworthiness of your partner. I'm much afraid that we may all have to get used to regular blood tests and to showing the results, on headed medical reports, to a new sexual partner. Come clean about past or present sexual infections and always sort them out quickly or you may be hated for causing suffering.

Being stoned will not bring satisfaction. Star lovers are never drunk or drugged, they just come fast and look stupid. Drunken women have little recall, no enjoyment and no control about cystitis, venereal disease or pregnancy. They look stupid, too.

Frigidity

Men rarely complain about frigid women now. Perhaps women enjoy sex more because they are better skilled or perhaps central heating means warmer rooms and warmer women. Divorce is a way out of very unreasonable behaviour. Women often feel the cold more than men but constantly pulling up bedclothes and wanting to wear a nightie, asking at intervals whether he's finished yet will quickly wreck the whole business! Pyjamas? Oh, for goodness sake!!

Cold Rooms

Sexual enjoyment in a cold room is a dead duck. If she's tight and dry in the vagina because she can't get warm, penetration will be trickier. It only needs three or four unsuccessful pushes at the vaginal entrance to increase vaginal resistance and damage ruining further pleasure. Increased penile pressure may tear the entrance, especially at the side nearest the back passage where the perineal seam is at its tightest and most resistant. Once there's a tiny tear, intercourse for that session will be mutually unpleasurable. She will be aware and thinking of every thrust and whether the tear will hurt or get worse. Hang the heating bill, turn the heating on!

Bacteria, if not previously washed off, will gain ready entrance through the tear and she may now face a twofold problem - the pain and soreness of the injury itself, plus infection. If this has happened before she'll also add fear to her trouble. It might range from two or three days of ordinary soreness - stinging on the tear as urine touches it - or it could go all the way to a big attack of bladder cystitis, not just urethral stinging. Any of this she will learn to dread.

Several months of such misery will remove thoughts of sex as a pleasure. Fear and dread of repeat cystitis will prevent intercourse! It doesn't take much imagination to understand far-reaching, long-term results of such trouble: sexual separation, distress, rows, doctors, investigations, separate bedrooms, sexual infidelity and total break up of the relationship. All from a cold bedroom I hear you say? Certainly, and the group most at risk are young lovers whose social conditions are less stable than in a homely place where heating can be controlled.

I had a young woman for counselling who was living with her boyfriend in his flat. He liked a cold bedroom and, being an economic guy as well, turned his heating off well in advance of bedtime. This meant that the bathroom was cold too. She survived the bedroom but couldn't pass urine or do bottle washing afterwards because the bathroom was too cold!

Her cystitis only ever happened after sex and lab tests on her urine sample showed positive infection, especially in wintry weather. Neither had fully acknowledged the tremendous importance of room temperatures. Once the place is warm, it becomes so much easier to change from one sexual position to another and to wash properly before and after intercourse.

The Bride's Disease

Honeymoon cystitis' or 'The Brides' Disease', as it was once called in the days when honeymoons were real, was purely caused by frequent, energetic penile thrusting into a tight, narrow vagina. Today, any sexual holiday can cause cystitis. You try banging your calf muscle with a broom handle for twenty minutes and see if it doesn't go pink, red or purple! You will also be going pink, red or purple inside, but it's impossible to see it. Rest for a second once inside to give the vagina time to 'recognise' the 'foreign' object and accept it.

Take a break!

If intercourse resumes before vaginal recovery, injury will be added to insult! Maybe total stoppage for two weeks! A racehorse doesn't run again the same day or even the next, it is rested! Neither does any sportsman !

Rest up afterwards if you are prone to twingeing after sex, don't put on trousers or jeans. Do plenty of cool water vaginal cleaning to reduce inflammation, drink lots of water and let tissues rest. Any sexual holiday or honeymoon can then continue happily unimpeded by cystitis.

Afterwards

Urine may sting as it runs down the urethra soon after intercourse but it will improve next time. Drink well. Swelling inside is not only confined to the vagina but will be affecting all sorts of places you wouldn't think of. With the urethral tube so close to penile thrusting, it too, goes into shock and swells. It stings when urine tries to flow down the gap between swollen urethral walls but you must pass urine and get the urinary system active quickly or waiting on will only worsen stinging later. Do a vaginal clean with very cool water after passing urine and return to bed or at least thirty minutes rest. Don't go walkabout wearing jeans, wear a longer skirt to allow cool air to circulate and drink water to replace lost body liquids.

Swollen skin outside and inside becomes a deep maroon or pale brown colour after a night's sleep. A night's rest and cool water vaginal cleaning is a vital help in reducing swelling even up to the battered cervix. By morning, soreness should have decreased unless intercourse has been more violent or prolongued when it may take longer.

The uterus (womb) may ache a little because the thrusting of the head of the penis onto the cervix may have involved the cervical canal and uterus. If you are close to a period the whole thing is more sensitive because uterine lining will already be heavy with gathered blood.

Intercourse During a Period

Intercourse at this time is naturally a bit messy, but it can also be helpful in easing period pain. It should be far gentler than normal with no deep positions and no heavy thrusting. Rhythmical relaxing and suctioning type movements can assist early congestion as blood tries to escape down the cervical canal into the vagina. Bear down gently at times and at others go quiet for a moment to feel the vagina open wider.

Put lots of dark towels on the bed, make sure the room is nice and warm so that all top bed clothes can be thrown off and not get spoiled. Intercourse at this time is an individual choice and many religions forbid it, but generally it takes place within a relationship of great intimacy, one that is totally committed to a love of each other's body. There are couples who adore intercourse at this time, and provided hygiene is very good and the bed carefully protected it can be blissful.

Orgasms

Don't always aim for the orgasm at the end. Young men can, over several hours of sex, have between two and four full ejaculations, so whilst you discover each other by watching and listening, make sure, too, that you look to the enjoyment of your own body, too. Female orgasms can vary between plateaux of gentle vaginal lubricants to matching, thrust for thrust and on to huge spurts of liquid from glands just inside the vagina. These are best achieved when the woman is on top and can ride off the penis to allow her liquid to come away, a penis tends to block it off. Bruising can also be limited because 'riding' controls depth of penetration.

Sex Sessions

Short, strong sexual sessions without stopping for a breather can cause awful bruising. The vagina must be allowed to stretch open once the penis is in it. Lengthy sexual sessions between experienced lovers have to be accompanied by interludes of talking, resting, drinking water and more lubricant gel. Position changing is really important here and so delightful! The vagina prefers well-spaced sex sessions but every woman knows what hers can put up with so do whatever happens naturally and healthily.

Urine will be building up because kidneys don't conveniently stop expelling it whilst you are making love! Don't hold it in because you're too embarrassed! Go and pass it! Afterwards, fill the mineral water bottle with very cool tap water, and, after passing urine, stay sitting on the lavatory whilst you pour the cool water down over the perineal openings. This water cools swollen skin and reduces inflammation. Pat dry gently and thoroughly and return for more! Drink water to replace lost fluids and use lubricant gel again before new penetration.

Energetic sex is one hell of an exercise! Both of you will be wonderfully sweaty and the bed quite damp. Take up a jug of iced water or orange squash, no juices and nothing too sweet in case thrush might be encouraged.

Theatricals

Use aromatherapy oils for gentle body stroking, drip wine or champagne on one another and lick it off or trickle it into one another's mouths- DON'T drink much because alcohol acidises urine and acts diuretically. Urine will be sparse and burn madly when you try to pass it afterwards. Many women are so sensitive that they have to choose between alcohol and sex. If you drink, don't have sex and if you choose sex one night forgo the alcohol, never mind don't drink and drive! Leave out coffee for the same reason.

The whole of the bed, its end and wall and its other three edges can all become theatrical props. You don't *have* to lie in a sleeping position of head at the top, feet at the bottom of the bed. You don't *have* to lie down at all! You can sit, kneel, bend over both on the bed and its edges. Flicking through just one copy of *Playboy* or *Penthouse* will spark off enough ideas for your own improvisation to last forever and most youngsters already have! Hard porn and bondage is very distasteful, often dangerous and quite unnecessary in happy sexual liaisons. You'll get far better kicks from your own inventions because being in a love/sex relationship, rather than just sex, is entirely your creation and your world. Porn films and magazines are not promoting love, they're promoting fortunes and slavery. Why make rich men richer?

What else?

It can be very exciting to have a man absolutely unable to control himself because he thinks you are sexy and gorgeous and he knows you can take it! If he is that excited, he'll probably be growing hard again in twenty or thirty minutes for a steadier and more prolonged intercourse. In the meantime have a good cuddle. Women love that and adore being held closely

All the following positions in the drawings (please note the central heating!) can be tried with care and yelled warnings if anything hurts! Dull, pleasurable ache is one thing, strong internal pain quite another. Sex, with health and cleanliness is the best possible sort of sex. Women have far more intercourse now than they used to years ago. That has to do with contraception, changed attitudes, warmer bedrooms, social intermingling and greater knowledge amongst other things. They need to stay well to enjoy it often.

Good, healthy, spaced sex is far better for everyone than smoking, drinking, drug-taking, workaholism, overeating, jogging, excessive keep fit classes. Healthy sex is good for the mind, decreases depression; is good for the body, keeps it supple; stops men straying quite so often! So enjoy it and value it because much can and does get in its way throughout life.

Sexual Non-bacterial Irritation and Bruising

Diagnosis
Apart from urine samples being well and truly negative, not even showing any plus signs (++) in the cell, pus, blood or protein boxes, nor any influence from a recent course of antibiotics or prior 'comfort' drinking, there remains another accurate way of helping to diagnose bladder irritation or bruising caused by intercourse as against true urinary infection.

Timing
Germs take 24 to 48 hours to exhibit symptoms, though I have seen very exceptional circumstances, such as the woman whose bacterial cystitis began 12 hours after sex, and the woman who did not present symptoms until 50 hours afterwards.

The 12-hour case was the result of using a bidet after diarrhoea and just before she was penetrated; in the 50-hour case a little (though ineffective) hygiene had been attempted. In the first case there was a heavy presence of coliform to start with; in the second case the presence was so low that it could only barely manage to stay active. But manage it did, with the 'help' of time, sex and an incomplete hygiene routine.

Mostly, sexually-activated bacterial cystitis will commence symptoms of an attack somewhere between 24 and 48 later, often without any intermediate signals at all.

In the case of non-bacterial irritation or bruising, however, soreness, swelling and inflammation can commence even during sex, building within hours to an attack, still without bacteria.

These signs of soreness disturb the urethral and bladder nerve endings during intercourse. They get 'excited', 'stimulated', 'upset' and react by telling you that urine needs to be passed. Minutes later, they repeat the demand, and then again and again.

What to Do?

Drink half a pint (10 fl. oz./250 ml) of water immediately and take three strong painkillers to block the 'excitement/stimulus'. Clean and calm the vagina with a lukewarm bottle wash and place a comforting hot-water bottle at your back. Drink a glass of water every 20 minutes until the bladder feels calmer or urine stops burning, or even do the Three-hour Management routine. Forget the sex!

What Could Have Caused It?

Full documentation of individual causes here is impossible. The circumstances of each woman's and each man's lovemaking are, of course, highly individual. All I can do is to give ideas and a few examples, to help you help yourself find the answer to your own problem. Was hygiene absolutely perfect for both partners? Female Bottle Washing and male showering?

TIMING: Look again at the timing.

Does your soreness or 'reaction' start before sex?

Can this be related to the contraceptive you are using. Could it be a pessary, a cream, a contraceptive foam, a contraceptive sponge, the lubricant on a female condom, perfume sprayed accidentally onto the inner labia when only a dab on each inner thigh was intended, uninformed and incorrect use of any soap on the vulva (vaginal/urethral openings); a hot bath rather than the recommended bottle washing procedure; a hot bubble bath; a swim or a session in the jacuzzi; a vaginal infection that you are pretending isn't there; depilatory cream on pubic hair; wrong use of an antiseptic or deodorant to disguise a strong odor; dry menopausal skin; sitting on a jean seam in the car all afternoon so the vulva is already restricted and bruised?

All of these, and probably many more, are set up by you, the owner of the poor vagina about to be further mistreated. No doctor is going to fathom out this sort of cause! You've got to!

Does soreness or 'reaction' start during sex?

I take an understanding of *'during sex'* to be any time from the first moment of foreplay of any sort, right through the duration of all sex acts, to stopping all genital/digital contact.

Again, can this be related to contraception? Often we stop quickly to insert or to put on barrier contraceptives. Does this cause an instant reaction? When the vagina is already warming up and blood vessels dilating, they may be more sensitive to creams and lubricants.

Oral/genital/hand contacts are minefields of prospective soreness. Think about beards, moustaches, 'designer stubble', strong tonguing, broken nails, dirty hands, insensitive finger work, one-spot only massaging, dildos, cucumbers, exotic condoms - you know the answer, no one else!

Size

Yes, he can be too big and too hard! Either let him ejaculate early (inside or out), or give him up! Once -the early ejaculation has decreased the hardness, try him again. Use a good lubricant jelly, not Vaseline, spittle, cuticle removal cream or anything else you feel like trying. Use a slow, gentle entry. Don't let him push and shove if it is hurting; try less penetrative positions and always change positions. Vaginas and bladders don't appreciate being pummelled in one place for half an hour (or longer!). If you sit on top, take control. just one thrust up from him when you are pushing down is an earth/moon collision, with cervical bruising a real possibility.

Any tearing of vaginal skin internally or at the entrance may split and bleed. You wouldn't rub a cut finger, so change position and protect the vagina, or else stop. Lubrication with a slow entry does reduce this problem significantly.

Surprisingly, short sex sessions, where pent-up emotions are a driving force and niceties are ignored, can traumatize and bruise more than sessions where slowness and gentleness over an hour might have appeared more likely to cause trouble.

Sex between real lovers isn't just genital; it is stroking, caressing, licking, talking, appreciating the music, communicating, experimenting.

Does your soreness or irritation start after sex?

All sorts of sex – except anal, violence or rape - are quite OK so long as real soreness or bruising do not occur. Every woman 'feels' the intercourse afterwards - a bit swollen and sensitive - it can be lovely in its way. Steps to calm it all down are easy and helpful.

Cool Water Bottle Washing Procedure (for after sex)

1. Go to a warm bathroom!
2. Wash hands and fill one or two 500-ml bottles with coolish water, not hot.

3. Sit on the toilet and pass urine.
4. Now do the pelvic tilt (backbone downwards).
5. From the front, slowly pour the tepid water down the perineum and clean off sexual secretions.
6. Insert the longest finger of your other hand and reach to the cervix, 'hooking out' more secretions, five or six times in and out as the water is trickling, so that this coolness cleans and calms the vagina. Use a second bottle, if needed. Inflammation will quickly lessen.
7. Stand up and pat dry with the wash-cloth kept for perineal drying.
8. Rest now! At least 10 minutes with your feet up and no underwear! Best of all, go to bed for a night's sleep. Drink a glass of water before you go.
9. Wash again in the morning. If your contraception prevents this, just wash down the outside.

Once all sexual activity has ceased, nothing more can actually cause soreness, bruising or irritation unless you stupidly take a hot bath, pull on a pair of jeans, go riding or even do a three-mile walk. The simple but incredibly effective cool water bottle wash stops all trouble.

Summary

So, sexually:

- A full bottle wash within one hour before sex cleans germs off and prepares the perineum. Follow it with a vaginal bottle wash if it is a bit 'stale' and finish with a lubricant.
- Passing urine, using the cool water vaginal bottle wash, resting and drinking prevents soreness/bruising after sex.

CHAPTER EIGHT

8 Sex in Pregnancy

Cystitis is no barrier to conceiving a child. If your cystitis is one of other symptoms suggesting hormone deficiencies, pelvic disorder, fallopian or ovarian obstructions then you wouldn't be likely to conceive anyway.

Neither Bacterial or Non-bacterial cystitis will stop conception but coping with continuing cystitis as well as the pregnancy, delivery, aftercare and a new baby may prove more stressful than anticipated.

Until pregnancy begins, body reaction is unpredictable. Pregnancy problems can range from nothing at all to increased nasal congestion, increased vaginal discharges, hemorrhoids, morning sickness, nausea, itchy thigh skin, swollen breasts, heartburn, glossier hair; no cystitis, less cystitis, more cystitis, first-time cystitis; urinary frequency, swollen ankles, increased sexual desire, decreased sexual desire, high blood pressure, and more individualities.

Genetics dictate embryonic development: hair colour for instance, skin sensitivity for instance, and physiological sensitivities. Lung and heart troubles, allergies and many diseases can be hereditary: could some forms of cystitis be hereditary? I have known grandmothers, mothers and daughters in one family develop it but there may be several reasons including same ineffective handed-down bathing patterns, favourite toiletries, clothes washing processes and of course, short perineums helping bacterial travel. Again, remember that cystitis is only a symptom of another basic condition. Hereditary tendencies can skip and even miss the opposite sex.

Neither of my grandmothers had honeymoon lifestyle conditions like mine. They never went swimming, would not have drunk wine with each meal, used no vaginal foam contraceptive, wore no nylon swimsuit, did not dehydrate the kidneys by sunbathing in Tunisian sunshine for two weeks. There would probably not have been lengthy sex sessions and they would certainly not have eaten hot spicy foodstuffs. I have no idea whether they contracted cystitis on their honeymoons but they may have done. I never asked because they were dead by the time I started asking questions.

My cystitis completely stopped in my first pregnancy (I didn't get it in my second one five years later, either, but by then I'd stopped the attacks myself outside of the pregnancy with self-help). At that time, neither myself or my doctors had a reason to offer for its disappearance and I just thanked God for nine months' relief. Between pregnancies, I returned to the same hellish state until seeing Mr. Shuttleworth when slowly, so slowly, I began to learn that I myself could take charge and prevent cystitis attacks. I thanked God for Mr. Shuttleworth, too, and his first mention of passing urine after intercourse which led on to all the other self help and prevention.

Pregnancy Discharges

Increased normal vaginal discharges during pregnancy irritate the urethral opening but can be easily cleaned out with a cool vaginal Bottle Wash. Increase bacterial vigilance with perfect bottle washing. Be especially careful about scrubbing fingers and nails before hooking out the discharge from the vagina. Again a reminder not to put any kind of soap on the vulva, but only plain water poured out of the bottle which will remove the itchy, but non-bacterial discharge and stop it being massaged up the urethra when you sit or walk. Go without underwear to keep the perineum dry and healthy and keep out of leotards, jeans and trousers.

If you get bacterial cystitis which has been properly diagnosed from a urine test, take the sensitive antibiotics prescribed, ask for vaginal pessaries to counteract any predisposition to vaginal thrush and eat three soup spoonfuls of live yoghurt twenty minutes before meals to encourage lactobacillus to fight full body thrush. Check the anal opening as you soap it during Bottle Washing when you can feel whether there are any hemorrhoids starting. Or are existing skin tabs and piles enlarging and increasingly attracting fecal germs?

Re-check all your actions after a bowel movement. If bowel movement patterns have altered, think about any effect from that, or maybe the stool is more frequent and almost diarrhoea. Are you washing after **each** movement? You must! Conversely, don't strain away when you are pregnant if the stool has become more solid. Take a safe laxative, eat stewed apples every other day and ask the pharmacist for a good anti-hemorrhoid suppository, or mention the problem to the doctor.

Bowels and bladder will be working for the two of you, so don't worry about passing more urine or more fecal material. Don't hold on and try not to let the bowels become congested or stools will be wider and more difficult to expel.

I know that since the thalidomide tragedy, pregnant women have been very scared of any drug, even if it's non-prescribable, but equally if you have an illness or infection in pregnancy and you let it spread untreated, this can be just as detrimental to the baby. Take what medication you must. Your doctor can allay fears on any pharmacological product so that you can enjoy your pregnancy.

From my work on mercury fillings, I possess dozens of papers and books about mercury in the endocrine system. It is truly shocking and my overwhelming advice is for prospective parents to rid themselves, safely, of ALL mercury fillings BEFORE attempting conception then the fetus is protected and breastmilk is uncontaminated. Mercury vapour exits through breastmilk just like nicotine, alcohol, drugs and general nutrition.

Intercourse

Go ahead. It must be made very plain to your husband that a shower each evening is great protection against vaginal infections or inflammations. Penetration from behind may be more comfortable, especially after the fourth or fifth month. Curl up and let him gently reach to a depth inside which you instinctively feel is not going to hurt either you or the baby. He should only use very gentle rhythmic pushing stopping at any discomfort signals from you. However, vaginal entry from behind carries with it the prospect of fecal residue coming off any piles onto the penis and into your vagina! Watch out!

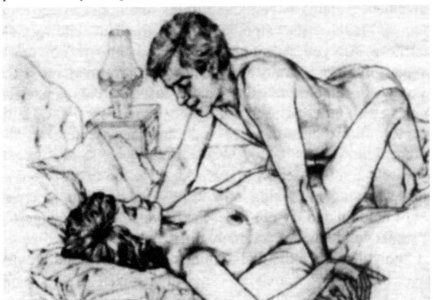

If you aren't too large yet, lie on your back, put one pillow in a position underneath you which will elongate your pelvis and let the baby move upwards with gravity to your waist out of the way! The penis can then move along the whole length of the vagina as he kneels between your legs and supports himself with sturdy arms. A few slow pushes and withdrawals of this kind with the baby between you will bring sheer joy. It's not enough movement to bruise or hurt the fetus.

Avoid strong orgasms or else risk miscarriage especially on period dates.

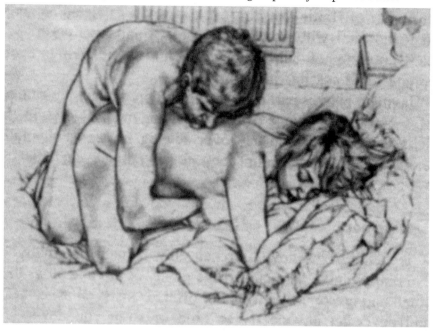

Sexual expressions change as pregnancy progresses towards birth. Usual acts of penetration alter but this a wonderful time to try new things and marvel at new life surging within you. Your bodies exist for the enjoyment of both of you, and you should both revel in nine months worth of extended arousal and freedom from contraceptive practices.

Second and subsequent pregnancies may renew old excitements but if you now bear scars including an episiotomy, these may affect lovemaking as skin once again stretches in later pregnancy. Lubricating gel is the key in such difficulties. Avoid bearing down either in orgasm, plateau orgasms, passing urine or passing fecal material.

Labour

A second episiotomy can make for much misery in bed and be an easy source of discomfort, trauma or infection. Discuss the scar with a good gynaecologist and try to avoid having it re-opened.

If you have a sensitive skin then refuse antibiotic swabbing in favour of Bottle Washing with a capful of Betadine taken in to hospital with you for use before and after birth. Salt baths, not too hot, help healing, too, and should help to avoid soreness and possible infections.

Having a baby is part of sex - the end product and beginning of a new era for your own body. Poor medical care in the delivery room, particularly over sewing up tears, internally and externally, can account for a never ending cycle of sexual misery.

Repairs

It is better right now to repair any damage internally or externally on the perineum. Take plenty of gas and air as they stitch and create a fuss if its not offered. Insist on anaesthesia and never let anyone try to hold or strap you down, it's barbaric! If you wriggle they can't stitch properly and future intercourse may be uncomfortable with an increase in infection so it's worth while having good pain reduction and quality stitching.

If after six weeks, the internal check-up shows jagged scars, flaps of skin, or loose stitching and there is discomfort, further surgery may be required.

Catheters

Bladder catheterisation should be avoided unless absolutely necessary but it is sometimes used during or after Caesarian sections when the bladder tries to re-start. Catheters invariably cause an attack of cystitis so insist on a full Bottle Wash before catheter insertion and wash three times a day until it is removed. Cystitis just may be avoided with this help but if it does start take prescribed, sensitive antibiotics and do the Three Hour Management procedure. The attack will go but be careful and insist on what I have said here.

In vaginal birthing, perineal skin can be strained to tearing point and an episiotomy may be preferable to untidy tearing which is more difficult to stitch up. Otherwise, let Nature and gravity take time for an unhurried delivery with minimal tearing.

Bacterial cystitis after delivery is not uncommon. Take your washing bottle to the hospital so that you can wash the perineum down just as though you were at home. After passing a stool, be very thorough so that anal bacteria can't get a hold in the damaged and bruised perineal skin. Make sure you line the hospital toilet seat in the front with paper so that infection risk is reduced.

Wear a loose sanitary towel, and if you are in bed don't bother to do it up over the pubic hair. Make sure that it is well placed at the back so that drainage is caught. If you lie with just the sheet over you and your legs bent, the perineum will cool and heal faster.

I'm not in favour of too many hot salt baths. The value of the salt is not denied, it's the doubtful value of the hot water when you are already swollen that I question. Bottle washing is still preferable so when you wash the perineum down after passing a stool pop some salt in the bottle for a final rinse off.

A Good Rest

Drink a fair amount to keep the bladder and urethra 'clean' and make every effort to excrete what you drink. Steer off sweetened drinks and juices except as real treats and watch out for all funny, yellow coloured drinks because the tartrazine doesn't agree with everyone. Too much "visitors" fruit like grapes, plums, strawberries etc., may acidize the urine and it will sting as it flows down a bruised urethra. Too much fruit will also give your baby diarrhoea if it's being breast-fed. Don't wear trousers, jeans or leotards anyway, this book should have warned you totally off them. The perineum needs air and coolness to heal from trauma and inflammation.

Later, very gentle exercises done on the bed will help flatten the abdominal muscles and tighten up the pelvic floor. They are important in preventing future prolapse of bladder and uterus. Prolapse operations, where they hitch up the bladder and/or the uterus, are never a hundred per cent successful and indeed the situation has to be quite bad in the first place before a surgeon will agree to operate.

If you have a good rest after a good delivery, and normality at home is returning, i.e. no discomfort on passing urine; no discomfort on passing a stool; no further bleeding; sitting on chairs with ease, it may be hard to wait for six weeks before resuming intercourse. Try to hang on until six weeks because the cervix and uterus may still be not quite back to size.

Resuming Intercourse

Lucky you, if intercourse feels alright when resumed after six weeks. The sheath and withdrawal may be the contraceptives best used for a while; plenty of gel, especially if you had an internal tear. Have a word with the gynaecologist at the check-up about contraceptives if you are breast-feeding. Some women go on the Pill once breast-feeding is secure but you are entitled to have your own ideas.

If there is no adverse discomfort, pain or urinary involvement perhaps childbirth suits you. The amount of time taken by individual women to recover their full sexual health is variable. Judge your improvement on a regular basis and try to gauge if the discomfort is lessening. If it is slowly decreasing, nature is simply taking time - no doctor can possibly improve on the natural healing process so be patient. Any discharge or bleeding should be reported and another internal given.

Once sexual intercourse is back to its previous patterns there will be opportunities for new positions, a sort of third phase. Tiredness may take the edge off the length of time you make love but it can stimulate new variations. Use lubricating gel if you're tired and dry to start with, and this will avoid aggravating any internal-bruising left over from the birth. Don't go off sex just because you may not feel as wet as you did before the baby. It'll come back once you are sexually psyched up.

Normality Returns

A recovered vagina after childbirth, provides greater depth and width for sexual positions. For instance, your husband may now be able to get three fingers inside and move them instead of just two; you might be able to bring both legs over his shoulders, an extremely deep entry and one which will become even more tolerable over the years as his rigidity declines. You may not yet feel like letting him move or thrust in this position, but wait on!

Sitting astride will still require guidance near menstruation, but halfway through the cycle should find you able to move on top comfortably. Once you're secure on top there are many simple enjoyments best left to other books or your own devising.

Toil and Memories

A heavy day at work may reduce erectile strength and it's this sort of occasion that lets you take a more active part. Use his body, he'll love that, freely exploring any deeply penetrative positions that would have produced discomfort before childbirth.

Memories of good or unusual intercourse unimpeded by sexual cystitis are part of the stuff of life. Remember them and store them for your old age when one of you is gone or sexuality no longer plays a part in life. Cystitis sufferers may find cystitis due to bruising and trauma, slowly decreasing over the years but the more sexual activity you have, the more likelihood there is of cystitis, urethritis, vaginitis and many other conditions. This is almost entirely controllable by prevention and self-help.

CHAPTER NINE

9 Sex in Later Life

The softer the penis becomes with advancing years the less chance there is of bruising and trauma in the female partner. 'Broomhandle' becomes a thing of the past. It widens although it doesn't necessarily lose length. Vaginal tone decreases because of menopause hormonal loss and infrequent intercourse. A softer penis and a shrinking vagina will not perform well either in duo or with other partners.

But for many sexually active people pleasure heightens because sex becomes more comfortable in middle age. After fifty, skill, co-ordination, less fear of pregnancy, mobility, more money and more leisure time give heightened sexual enjoyment if sexual machinery is in good shape.

The whole range of sexual positions becomes possible, though perhaps stale marriages, weary from child-rearing and career commitments, are not so conducive to a good romp. Revitalize your life with some mineral supplements, some weight reduction and maybe a treat week at a health farm. Go shopping for a new set of underwear and new sheets or take a weekend away, whatever might turn you both on.

The most common sexual cause of cystitis is infection but equally, soreness can cause misery in later years. Main proof comes again from urine samples and vaginal swabs. As vaginal health begins its gradual decline near, during and after menopause, the lining may become more prone to invasive bacteria and to dryness but there is much that can be done to counteract it with HRT and self help.

HRT- Hormone Replacement Therapy

Dryness is treatable. Simple sexual dryness will respond to lubricating gel, but if the dryness is bordering on continual discomfort or burning, hormone treatment may be indicated. Other symptoms of hormone imbalance include depression, lethargy, hot flushes, limb aches, cystitis and great vaginal discomfort. Some women only need occasional smears of vaginal hormone cream to keep a healthy vagina ready for intercourse, but others may have to investigate stronger treatments. In severe menopausal problems experiments with conventional tablets, implants and injections, natural hormone treatments like Red Clover; any may provide better relief.

Find a menopause clinic or a gynaecologist whose life's work centres upon this area of women's health. Improvement in attitude is happening but it's slow, though research shows big improvements in osteoporosis and heart problems as decreased estrogen levels rise again on treatment.

Most patients experience improvement in quality of life and symptoms. Patience and monitoring produce results. Severe menopausal problems can disappear if mercury amalgams are safely removed.

Libido

Libido should improve once vaginal burning and discomfort wane. Work on vaginal acceptance of penetration with a week of foreplay and a soft dildo. Start with a small one then move up the scale until one approximating to your partner's size is reached. Real intercourse can start carefully with plenty of jelly so that sex can be enjoyed perhaps twice-weekly. The more the ageing vagina is used the healthier it will be. Regular intercourse is effective in counteracting ageing and both partners need to work at sexual maintenance.

The world of erectile dysfunction is not so secretive since the arrival of Viagra. This extraordinary drug is an enormous improvement for common erection problems and has now encouraged many manufacturers to research non-medical types of treatments. Herbal and natural products can be tried and Viagra itself can be prescribed or bought on the web. Prices will decrease eventually.

Mercury influence

I should also add that mercury vapour from teeth fillings may disrupt hormones at any age especially menopause because by then there may be a mouthful of fillings, caps and bridges. Better still, don't let it get to this stage, have white composite fillings but not the glass ionomer type. See a mercury-free dentist and get as much poisonous metal out as reasonably and safely possible. Menopausal problems may then very well decline as they did in my case. Erection problems can also disappear with safe mercury removal as the testes, glans and shaft recover strength. Chelation processes are designed to expel and excrete lifelong stored mercury from all organs.

Marriage supports young, middle and old years together so that age creeps on slowly and with dignity. If the overall relationship stays happy, sexual happiness should go hand in hand, with intercourse remaining as one part of that overall happiness. Life isn't like that, though, for the majority, and such ideals are very hard to achieve. If doctors have to step in with replacement therapy to stop aches, pains and more severe symptoms like cystitis we should all be grateful that at least such therapy does exist.

Old Age

Sex in old age is only possible if vaginal skin is kept in good tone; the oldest woman I knew of still fairly sexually active was 84 years, but once intercourse stops for good, the vagina practically closes up shop. Muscles collapse, the tube itself collapses and even a doctor's finger inserted for examination may meet with defeat. Skin is almost opaque and incredibly thin. Nevertheless, cystitis and infections can still create real hell and hormone cream may improve comfort even if only smeared along the perineum with a gentle finger.

Cystitis at this late stage is obviously not primarily sexual, it can be caused by thin skin, possibly higher sugar levels, fungal infections and an inability to practise efficient perineal hygiene. Care homes, nursing homes and geriatric hospitals are full of it.

CHAPTER TEN

10 Other Sorts of Sex

This book is not written to moralize. It is written to help people achieve happy, safe, healthy sexual intercourse. Enough has already been told of the inherent dangers of sexual infections and I ask everyone to keep their wits about them and stay healthy.

Rape

Rape as a cause of cystitis will now make sense to the reader but it has not always been obvious. Rape crisis centres and forensic police doctors recognise cystitis and awful urethral and bladder damage from violent penetration. The victim's age is immaterial. That she may be skilled and well practised at breathing deeply and expanding her vagina counts for nothing in the state of panting fear induced by threatened and real physical violence.

At every turn the victim's fear produces immense tension in the pelvis and that tension removes the elasticity necessary for internal organs to slide out of the way of an incoming object. Damage to bladder, uterus, cervix and bowel will vary according to the violence of the entry and thrust. Damage to the perineum will be really bad with general body bruising around the waist.

Street rape may be of shorter duration than rape in a quieter place since fear of discovery is greater. It may be accompanied by a knife threat to subdue the victim faster without the need for using his own arms and legs in the overpowering.

The victim's dilemma is that resistance may increase injuries. If there's really no way out and you haven't learnt any self-defence, talk. Talk and co-operate to calm the situation a bit if possible. Remain as still as you can under what are appalling circumstances. If two men are at it, the second may be easier because the ejaculate from the first will act as a lubricant. Above all else protect your life.

When it's over go to the police immediately. Don't go home. Ring a door bell and ask for help. Stay on the doorstep unless an obviously reliable person answers. Remember all you can and fix relevant details in your mind. Don't wash, not even your hands. If you managed to scratch him, there could be valuable evidence under your nails of his blood group, tissue, hair and semen. These may also be on your clothes, underwear and perineal skin. Mentally log as many details as possible.

Only when the police doctor has taken full swabs, tests and visual evidence should you shower, bath, Bottle Wash and change, unless you are hospitalized.

Then put into action the Management of an Attack of Cystitis. Use plenty of cool bottled water on genitalia. Bed rest will help a lot if you are not recommended for hospital, but even there, cooling air and cool water wash-downs will aid tissue healing enormously. Take Arnica to help reduce internal inflammation or else strong anti-inflammatory tablets.

It may take several days, or a couple of weeks for soreness and bruising to go. During that time urinary or vaginal infection will start, if they are going to. More swabs and a urine test are essential to reveal any bacteria and to treat it accurately. A general broad-spectrum antibiotic may not be sensitive to the specific bacteria found in the samples, hence the accurate testing.

It may be well worthwhile to start talking straightaway to a psychotherapist. Better to have the trauma out now than let it seep into your brain and cause years of anguish.

If you are desperately unfortunate enough to have serious internal organ damage, you may need a really first-class gynaecologist, urologist and proctologist (for the bowels) and tremendous courage and perseverance.

Sex For Handicapped People

Paraplegics or tetraplegics, people with disabling diseases, people who have external bags instead of bowel or bladder are all still able in some way to make love. Account is taken of the disability, of course, but cuddling, handwork and a variety of penetration positions are perfectly possible.

That being so, all the usual preparations for healthy intercourse are still required. Scrupulous penile and perineal hygiene is mandatory. However, depending on the impaired mobility, it can be difficult or even impossible to go to a strange toilet set-up before intercourse. Where washing before intercourse may take able-bodied people twenty seconds or, conversely, be part of foreplay, so for the disabled person who has to be lifted on to a toilet and washed, such activity can decidedly wreck the atmosphere of sexual arousal. When bowels are opened manually the disabled person performs careful hygiene then and tends to make that do for the day. All I am recommending here is that should urinary or vaginal problems tend to arise after sex then do revise and re-think your hygiene.

It is quite incredible that internal organs all work despite paralysis; urine is still manufactured by the kidneys; blood still flows; digestion still breaks food into micro particles and the uterus can still grow babies. Its amazing really.

Contraception, therefore, needs discussion and experiment. Adverse reactions to contraceptives are just as likely to lead to urethritis, vaginitis and cystitis. Infection, although painless, can still result from intercourse and kidney involvement can become a real danger. Urinary retention harbours infection and encourages bladder bruising during intercourse.

There is much reading material for disabled and injured people so go and search for ideas.

CHAPTER ELEVEN

11 Summary

Sexual cystitis even in its mildest, most temporary form is experienced by nearly every woman when starting to have intercourse. 'Honeymoon' bruising escapes very few and if ineffective hygiene allows bacteria to penetrate the bruised, raw skin then a miserable, painful week will ensue.

My main aim in life is to let women know how to avoid such misery. For heaven's sake, show this book to any woman, younger or older, who confides such a problem. To suffer for years, as I did, and many millions more women even longer before my work began, must now become a thing of the past. I lecture to any group and will counsel one-to-one if you really can't sort yourself out from these pages.

I want women to have as much sex as possible. Sex is very good for you and your partner, if you care for the organs used in the proper and appropriate way. If this book is a great help to women then it must also be an eye opener for men, so hand it to yours as well and maybe he'll pick up a few tips. Perhaps he'll even start a discussion on his rating as a lover!

Having lost so much of my own sexuality from my years as a cystitis and thrush victim, I realize that I could have prevented those particular years had I known what I know now. I am quite determined that you don't suffer like that.

BOOK THREE

Interstitial Cystitis

CHAPTER ONE

1 Symptoms and Diagnosis

What exactly is it?

Inter	means	*between*
stitial	means	*layers*
cyst	means	*sac, pouch or bladder*
itis	means	*inflammation and/or infection*

ALL THE PHRASE REALLY MEANS IS:

Some kind of inflammation and/or infection between the layers of bladder tissue.

So it is not some excitingly new and rare disease, but it is certainly utterly misunderstood by the medical profession which shakes its head, mystified, informing each sufferer at the end of the day, that nothing can be done to cure it. But then the medical profession is often mystified!

The main symptoms are fairly simply described although varying in intensity. *All real IC victims suffer 24 hour bladder pain, seven days a week and urinary frequency.*

Some days may be better than others leading to endless lifestyle investigations and examinations. Life is suspended for many since varying pain and frequency dominate all other activity and work prospects.

Bladder granulation and ulceration is often a final medical pronouncement confirming IC.

At this point professionals seem pleased with themselves and offer weekly bladder installations of RMSO to lessen the pain. They offer no curative treatments. And this is because they have none, nor any idea what it is that they need to cure!

Where is all this disaster beginning and what really is the cause? Because until this is known no firm treatment can begin and no real hope of cure can be entertained. Cause or causes are the most basic investigative and diagnostic objectives in bladder detective work.

The first two books of this Encyclopaedia show the enormous number of personal reasons for individual attacks of cystitis, literally thousands branching out into every home along main investigative paths of lifestyle. Much so called IC is misdiagnosed by lazy professionals and inefficient laboratories.

American Work

Dr Larrian Gillespie in the States wrote a book about IC some years ago now but she mainly offered self help which plays a lesser role in the actual treatment of IC, though not its prevention and I disagree with much of her theory and postulations. It is also true to say that most urologists have jumped on a bandwagon frequently just saying that a patient with ordinary cystitis has IC. This is not acceptable either, it's a misdiagnosis. The main question governing diagnosis of IC is this:

Do you have unremitting pain 24 hours a day, seven days a week without any breaks whatsoever and have frequency most of the time?

If the answer is firmly **YES**, then I accept that you may have this condition called Interstitial Cystitis. If bladder biopsies show granulated, reddened patches or ulcers then I am even more convinced but I would want to **SEE** that diagnosis in writing! It is not good enough just to be told it. It may be part of the big medical fob-off! Get it in writing! Get a second opinion!

In fact **ASK** to see your notes. Americans are able to hold their own notes which, of course, enables them be seen and allows safe-keeping. In the National Health Service of the United Kingdom patients do now have the right to see notes but not the right to hold them safely at home. Many notes go astray in this system.

When I began my work on cystitis in 1971 women were told that they had the Urethral Syndrome, with unknown causes and no cures! It was a massive medical fob-off and excuse to proceed no further with any detective work. It also showed how ignorant the professionals were and largely still are. My self-help work stopped diagnostic reliance on the "Urethral Syndrome" and offered all the self help required to prevent any more attacks of cystitis. I want to stop similarly muddled, false and ignorant medical pronouncements on IC.

Frequent dilations by zealous urologists, especially in America, will have scarred the urethral tube also the Trigone, which is just inside the bladder, and may probably have damaged the bladder wall as well. Into all this scarring will come more bacteria because it is now weakened tissue. It will over time and more dilations lose muscle tone so some level of incontinence or dribbling may add to your woes. The urologist also, will have added to your woes and you or your insurers will have added to his pockets!

We know that IC has proved an intractable problem to patients and doctors alike. It is a far worse problem in the States because of misleading information, ineffective laboratory work and too much urethral dilation practised there. Dr Gillespie's book in the early 1990's on IC stated clearly that :

"IC is NOT due to bacteria, like cystitis, but is a complex syndrome boiling

down to how many ways can you deprive bladder tissue of oxygen by altering blood flow".

She states also that:
"The poor bladder is only a messenger for a problem occurring elsewhere in the body".
I think of the bladder as a receptacle, not a messenger and as such receives the results of lifestyle such as sexual bacteria, poor hygiene, alcohol binges, chemicals and low liquid intake (see elsewhere in this Encyclopaedia for countless other contributions).
Her distinction between the two types of cystitis, presumably between IC and normal attacks, is:
"IC is cramping, burning and pressure relieved BEFORE and AFTER urination, while cystitis is the same thing WHEN you urinate"!!
I find this difficult to understand. Severe attacks of 'normal' cystitis can and do cause painful urination for the duration of the attack and there is pain whether passing or not passing urine.
Although this doctor was the first to write about IC, her ideas were as inconclusive as many contemporary doctors and many desperate women sought alternative therapies that served to drain their bank accounts. Curing the problem of IC failed to happen.
Another doctor, Dr Paul Fugazzotto in America, has reportedly found enterococcus in bladder urine samples of hundreds of desperate women. He takes far longer to culture a urine sample by using a culture 'broth' over several hours rather than the normal short lab system on a culture dish. This has had apparent success in 'most' of his patients by finding the 'sensitive' antibiotic appropriate to the specific bacteria discovered.
Now, this may simply be taking care of many incorrectly diagnosed patients with 'ordinary' cystitis where other labs had completely failed in conjunction with poor patient complicity in sample preparation. **It is no good drinking before taking the sample or having taken antibiotics in the previous 2-3 weeks for anything at all, or taking the sample in on a Friday afternoon. Urine must be concentrated, fresh and unhindered by recent antibiotics.**
A research project is currently underway by a team of neurobiology scientists in Virginia assessing Dr. Fugazzotto's broth culture process in relation to patients who have had no success in finding pathogens by any other means. This culture broth process has in fact been in use in prime research units since the 1980's so its actually nothing new but since most labs accepting urine for culture use a different method, Dr Fugazzotto's action may indeed be unusual. The Virginia

research is probably money and time mis-spent, the science is already proven elsewhere.

It is time to take the lid off Interstitial Cystitis and sadly once again show up urology for what it largely is - a time-wasting, money grabbing, uneducated branch of the medical profession when it comes to women's cystitis problems. Urological surgeons are only taught to operate and to perform theatrical or surgical diagnostic procedures such as urodynamics, cystoscopies, dilations and scans. They seem incapable of thinking about whether the infection/inflammation is a lifestyle reaction and later working out a lifestyle change to suit the circumstances and prevent recurrence.

British Work

Interstitial Cystitis is not initially about lifestyle changes, it is about Mycobacteria for which doctors scorn requests for laboratory testing, and laboratories which may not even have the test bench set up. Hardly any facilities exist in the United Kingdom and I am uncertain of the situation in the States. But, because Mycobacteria are already part of the flora and fauna of genitalia, as indeed are many other bacteria, all the professionals think its normal anyway. So no-one bothers testing for it and patients are kept utterly in the dark even about its existence. One never sees it on a swab or urine report!! Unless of course, you know me or the people I know!!

All the distressed women coming to me for counselling with the main symptom of unremitting pain 24 hours a day, seven days a week show a heavy presence of Myco bacteria of some sort in their tests and all respond to the specific antibiotic that gets rid of it; only one antibiotic works well and that must be taken in a very large VD dose dependent upon the number of years suffering.

I say that IC originates as a Sexually Transmittable Disease either by genital or oral / genital contact. It only needed the one initial contact perhaps many, many years ago, to set up a colony of Mycobacteria and cause years of pain, distress, hospital appointments to no avail, job loss, fights with medical authorities and social authorities for lost income, lost relationships and loss of life quality. We know that Mycobacterium tuberculosis can be found in the bladder because scientific studies have shown plenty of it. I maintain that in IC the medical profession is not looking for other forms of Mycobacteria and Ureaplasma urealyticum in bladder urine samples and biopsies nor in vaginal swabs and biopsies.

"Ureaplasma and Mycoplasma as a group of organisms are the least investigated and are probably the cause of more chronic urinary and gynaecological problems than any class of bacteria. They should be considered as a cause of cases of I.C. in women and Non Specific Urethritis in men. They may also be a causative organism in Bacterial Vaginosis and vaginitis thought to be caused by Candida." Dr Fred Lim, Consultant in Genito Urinary Medicine.

But we are going to look carefully at all this and then learn how to defeat difficult bacteria.

CHAPTER TWO

2 Unusual Bacteria

Enterococcus

WHAT IS IT?

It is a cell shaped bacterium originally thought to be a Streptococcus when found in the early 1900's. But in the 1930's Streptococcus fecalis was re-classified as Enterococcus because it was found to be able to grow at 100 Centigrade (450 Fahrenheit). Various technical laboratory improvements have now divided Strep fecalis into three groups: Enterococcus, Lactococcus and Streptococcus. Strep fecalis and Strep fecium, all originating in the bowels, were re-designated as Enterococcus fecalis and Enterococcus fecium in 1984. Several new species have arrived since then.

HABITAT

Enterococci are to be found in everyone's intestines, in all animal life and even on some plants. This means that they exit from the bowels in feces just like the bacteria discussed elsewhere.

They are apparently less frequently found in the vagina, mouth or dental plaque but of course, are abundant in sewage. Since they produce Lactic Acid they are often used in cheese production and can be found on cheeses, some meats and other food categories. Intestinal food sources create a perfect environment for production and reproduction of hundreds of bacterial variants and when those of the main groups exit in feces or diarrhoea, bacterial transfer to the urethral opening is easy. General moisture on the female perineum, walking around and all manner of sexual / oral intercourse transfer enterococci to welcoming sites.

TRANSMISSION

Between 1986 and 1989, Enterococcus was shown in studies to be the second most common cause of urinary tract infections and wound infections. It spreads via contact and is transmissable person to person both in the bedroom, bathroom, on plates, through drug abuse, in hospitals and from medical staff failing to wash their hands between patient's examinations. Catheters, dilations, laparoscopies, bowel examinations, cystoscopies and over use of antibiotics all encourage transmission. It is increasingly seen in older men with prostatitis probably because of inefficient hand and foreskin hygiene. Mothers no longer circumcise baby boys or teach foreskin retraction to clean properly and men, unlike women, fail to use sufficient toilet paper or wash hands.

Enterococcus is also seen in the newly born caused again by instrumentation, poor hygiene and low immunity with premature babies being particularly at risk. Pelvic infections, endometriosis, salpingitis, caesarian wound infections and peritonitis can all be caused by colonisation with Enterococci. There are now over a dozen species of Enterococcus isolated from plants and animals including humans but between 85 and 95% are of the E. fecalis variety.

IDENTIFICATION

E. fecalis and E. fecium can be readily identified from commercial tests but the variants and less frequently found varieties need stricter laboratory handling. The average laboratory whether State or private is not commercially keen on expensive outlays for less frequently observed bacteria. However these are not those most often found in cystitis so it becomes far more difficult for a patient and doctor to discover the precise variant and its sensitive antibiotic.

This is apparently where Dr Fugazotto is making his mark in America. He uses broths to culture samples in greater detail. These broths are based on acid formation in E. species and have to vary because E. strains vary and show up in different broths. The three broths used world-wide are mannitol, sorbitol and sorbose. A urine sample with an as yet unknown Enterococcus, may need to be cultured for certainty in each of these broths. This work is unavailable in practically every laboratory. Even so, researchers know and use these broths for scientific purposes and broth culture techniques ought to be more readily available in commercial labs.

APPROPRIATE ANTIBIOTICS

Because Enterococci have been exposed so frequently to broad spectrum antibiotics they have genetically altered and become resistant. **Intrinsic** resistance comes from inherited chromosomal changes but **acquired** resistance happens when existing bacterial DNA mutates into a different form. Intrinsically resistant E. strains are resistant to cephalosporins and some penicillins. Acquired resistance E.strains are more resistant to tetracycline, chloramphenicol and erythromycin. E. fecium is found to be resistant to vancomycin and more worryingly, the glycopeptide group of antibiotics.

The best guess antibiotics in common strains of Enterococci are still reckoned as ampicillin, penicillin or vancomycin, these are the ones tested in culture for sensitivity, i.e. sensitivity = will kill or inhibit bacterial reproduction.

Enterococcus can also cause serious systemic infections and treatment is therefore stronger and more prolongued in such cases, sometimes in Endocarditis treatment mixed antibiotics are prescribed.

OUTCOME

All reference books make pleas for greater hygiene in the control of Enterococci. Taking constant antibiotics causes resistant strains to emerge leaving physicians with little or no choice of antibiotics. Such books go so far as to suggest perineal swabbing or washing with hexachlorophene or chlorhexadine solutions. This is not the long-term answer nor the safe one. Chlorhexadine causes serious inflammation of the genital area after two or three swabbings and will initiate its own version of cystitis or urinary tract inflammation. Urethral, rectal and vaginal skin will either immediately or eventually swell, itch and burn, shortly causing internal inflammation as well.

The answer is to take the appropriate antibiotics as indicated by culture BUT then to initiate the full Bottle Washing procedure as previously directed each morning, after passing a stool, before all sorts of sexual intercourse and last thing at night. This simple effective hygiene must last for life until you die. All bowel bacteria will be washed out of harm's way regularly preventing new hourly bacterial transference.

It is worth wagging a finger again for correct sample taking.

Taking a clean sample
1. Clean off the vulval area with a wet cotton wool swab.
2. For Mycoplasma. Pass the first part of the urine flow into a sterilised container and the remainder into the toilet. This gives a more concentrated sample. More bacteria can be isolated giving a positive result rather than infuriatingly 'insignificant' or 'negative'.
3. Pour the sample into a sterile sample jar given by the doctor or even bought from a pharmacy and get it to the correct lab quickly.
4. Regular urine samples should be refrigerated until morning or when you know the collection van is due at your surgery.
5. Make certain it is refrigerated at the surgery and not put under the desk or on the window sill!
6. Even discuss taking it to the lab yourself or giving the sample there if its a long journey.

7. Don't bother after Friday lunchtime until Monday morning!! It will just sit around going off!

Taking a correct sample and obtaining the proper result is not just down to the lab it is a definite partnership between you both. Whether what I have written here makes you think about your part in all your 'insignificant' or negative' results over many years may suggest trying again locally especially if you do get 'breaks' between bad times or cystitis attacks. Whatever the strain of enterococcus, if it turns out to be that anyway, it is all down to you not washing off fecal residue or wind-blown fecal spores. Or if not you, then your sexual partner's unclean foreskin and poor hygiene habits. **Remember, Enterococcus is only a re-name of some types of Streptococci** and most of us have had Streps in our urine causing cystitis at some time until we knew when and how to Bottle Wash.

Dental Infections

Because this section on IC discusses unremitting infections with ongoing symptoms, all possible causes are important to relate. IC is certainly due to infection from somewhere of some sort and so we cannot discount rarities. Links between dental infection and the bladder becomes very obvious when you understand that the bladder is a receptacle at the end stage of urinary excretion. Whichever bacteria find a way either down into it or up, from an external source, may be important to someone struggling to find an answer.

If you have influenza, urinary excretion rates for the first few hours increase. Drinking plenty helps kidneys to flush out the systemic virus and keep pace with the increased excretion of urine. We all know this. Similarly, victims of severe mercury poisoning often have urinary frequency, usually without any pain, for weeks until the acute overload starts decreasing. This happens after dental fillings placement when the mercury already in situ has another load of poison dumped into the mouth. Immune system lymphocytes rush around encouraging excretion of mercury which is also well known as having diuretic properties. It was in use as a diuretic for years. So dental work with mercury can cause frequency, how about actual bacterial infection?

Oral Staphylococcus

This group of bacteria as described in the first segment of this book is also present in the mouth, most particularly under root canal treated teeth. A denervated tooth is dead, only some of its dentin tubules remain as obvious structure but inside there is now no blood or nerves. Metal posts, various cements and then a gold alloy under porcelain or a plain gold crown allow the 'structure' to be saved. BUT immune response is to sweep up and dispose of this dead item perceiving it as a threat to whole body health. Lymphocytes, phagocytes and the like try desperately and unceasingly to get rid of it. When they fail colonies form under, around and within this dead structure because they are not programmed to stop! Nature does just the same to an injured limb when gangrene sets in, the limb may need cutting off to save life! A dead, poisoned tooth needs the same treatment.

If not, the bacterial process remains ongoing and at some point an abscess will form, it will certainly form! You can scream from this pain. After many years of the dentist cleaning out and replacing the metallic supports, bacteria and their highly poisonous chemical toxins start to migrate into gum and jaw tissue. This is also called granulation when healthy tissue is attacked and breached. The process has been known for more than half a century to cause systemic ill health. Such a dead tooth and its toxins can transfer bacteria to all sorts of other sites in the body. Obviously the bladder as a receptacle will also receive this hazardous material.

Over time, bladder walls may become inflamed and sore, attracting colonies of dental bacteria if the offending jaw tissue or dead tooth is not removed. Most dental infections are Staphylococcus but not all. Ulcerated areas may start to redden and granulation tissue develops. If genital hygiene is wonderful but urine tests show inexplicable Staph infections look to the mouth and use the diary to look back for root canal treatments or very deep filling placements. Did cystitis or frequency start straightaway or a few weeks later? Just one tooth can cause trouble.

So many people never examine their mouth. Find a mirror and look in. Count up the fillings and caps/crowns. Don't have dental implants either, all that poisonous metal unnaturally embedded in jawbone!!! Have extractions when a tooth dies and, when too many are dead for you to be healthy or to chew happily, have the whole lot out. What we really want is genetic ability to re-grow our own teeth, this should prove far safer! But for now, systemic health is being compromised by keen dentists lining their pockets with repeat Root treatments!

In the 1920's the famous Dr Weston Price in America performed thousands of rabbit experiments using extracted human teeth replaced in the necks of thousands of rabbits. The rabbits showed the identical human ailments and bacterial presence becoming equally ill. Many died from overwhelming infections and Dr Price did a good number of experiments on bladders and kidneys. He took thousands of photographs and meticulously recorded every observation so that no doubt could be cast on his science.

He showed many bladder ulcers and urinary infections resulting from rotting, staph-diseased teeth. In human urine bacterial samples the infections of teeth that were causing abscesses and pain matched exactly and became identical in rabbits. In my experience, I have not specifically looked for nor counselled anyone like this, although some have seemed to correlate with dental treatments.

Doctors will find this hard to understand but look into your own diary and see if you can trace any link. Certainly Staphylococcus is found in many urine samples and if there has been no sexual activity at all for years with Staph being returned in the urine samples regularly, teeth might be the root cause.

Mycoplasma

Although the first Mycoplasma was discovered in the 19th century it was not until the 20th that the first urogenital example was seen under microscopy. The colony was so tiny that it was then called a T-strain but the group is now known universally as ureaplasma. In 1981 Taylor and Robinson, two researchers in University College named the first Mycoplasma genitalium from a closely observed specimen and from this several others all associated with the urogenital tract have been discovered and named.

FEATURES

These organisms are so small that they even lack a cell wall. Like miniscule jellyfish, they constantly alter shape and are difficult to verify even with modern culture technology. Only in the late 1980's with Polymerase Chain Reaction technology was M. genitalium able to be assayed. Mycobacteria glide rather than swim or cluster up together and because they are so slim many antibiotics simply cannot bind to them. They are usually anaerobic, not needing oxygen, but the commonest, Urea urealyticum and Mycobacterium hominis, don't mind air contact and are nutrified with sugars, arginine and urea.

SYMPTOMS

They have an ability to adhere to cells on vaginal and urethral walls and leave a very sticky, profuse discharge on underwear or pubic hair. Smegma on and under the foreskin provides perfect conditions of air, moisture and warmth from which oral and genital intercourse transfer colonies into the mouth, vagina and urethral opening. Other symptoms apart from the profuse, glooey discharge include itching, redness, pain locally or in the general pelvic region, period-type aches, general malaise if its in the bloodstream, backache and perhaps a heavy head.

Mycoplasmas tend to inhabit lungs, as in M.pneumoniae, M.salivarium, M. orale, and also urogenital tracts, as in

M. hominis, M.ureaplasma, M.genitalium. Lungs and genitals are warm, moist and enriched with foodstuffs. Lungs may also breathe in the fecal residue of oral sex. Kidneys may be on the receiving end also as swallowed smegma and fecal particulate reaches both intestines and kidneys via bloodstream and stomach. Oral intercourse tends to cause pelvic and back twingeing rather than full-blown urethritis and cystitis particularly in a 'young' episode. As the organisms gather speed more sites become infected and the symptoms deepen.

TESTING AND CULTURES

Samples for biopsy MUST only be taken from sites where cells have colonised or presumably from where the vaginal wall looks most red. Such areas contain the greatest adhesion sites affording the best opportunity for a positive result. Successful bladder biopsies can also show Mycoplasma when taken from a reddened, granulated site on the bladder wall. This has been done in London. Such a site may also be associated with ulceration. Ulcerated areas should be tested for Mycoplasma and U. urealyticum.

In culture these two genital infections require greater care and dark-field or phase-contrast microscopy should be used with temperature set between 360 and 380 Centigrade. They can be grown on a blood agar plate but for over six hours because they are very slow growers penetrating into the agar so that they look a bit like a fried egg. In a broth culture U. urealyticum may only take one hour to grow but M.genitalium and M.hominis may take six hours. The culture medium is complicated and includes several ingredients including yeast extracts, horse serum, blood, glucose and others.

For any lab or doctor wishing to set up a bench for Mycoplasmas, methodology is to be found in "Principles and Practice of Clinical Biology", published by John Wiley, 1997, pages 715-716 where the author of this section, Christiane Bebeare, advocates fastidious quality control because Mycoplasmas are so difficult to find otherwise.

A fast lane way of diagnosing the presence of mycoplasma is suggested as looking for antigens. This blood test looks for the immune system response to a previous or current presence of antibodies that have already come into contact with and fought the invading infective organism. Antibodies maintain a memory of it by simply being present in the blood. However, this is not a perfect detection and may not allow a technical infection to be reported by the laboratory microbiologist. The Report may return as Insignificant or No growth. Broths remain the favourite medium for attempting to culture mycobacteria and mycoplasmas.

Throat, oral and nasopharyngeal swabs can also be collected and cultured for these organisms but sputum is largely unsuccessful. Genital mycoplasma samples can be taken from semen, first-void urine, prostatic secretions, urethral swabs, endometrial biopsies, bladder biopsies, tubal brushing, amniotic fluid, placenta. Cerebrospinal fluid, blood and synovial fluid are some of the other possible sample aeeas.

Vaginal presence of U. urealyticum may be found in 50% of the female population, but M.hominis only in 15%. Interestingly, mycoplasmas in conventionally taken urine samples may often be reported as 'contaminated sample'! How many of us have had that down on the sample report! Most doctors would read that as the patient not having swabbed properly before taking the sample. If this happens to you ask for a repeat sample insisting that the doctor specifically asks for Mycoplasma testing! Remember to take the first part of the flow! This is where colonisation is strongest.

Remember also to check for a lab near you that can test for Mycoplasmas at all! They are few and far between and you may have to travel! Try to arrange for onsite testing in this case as samples must be fresh without storage at all.

Mycoplasmas may well be the causative organism behind the ubiquitous Bacterial Vaginosis and indeed, I had that diagnosis off two State swabs before insisting on a private clinic swab for Mycoplasma. It turned out to be M.hominis and I'd had it for at least three years! Of the seven known genital mycoplasmas, Urea urealyticum and M.hominis are very commonly found in the general population probably giving rise to medical and laboratory **dis**interest. Even if the lab sees evidence of colonisation they may well not be reporting it back because it is regarded as normal flora.

M.hominis has been found present in cases of pyelonephritis, kidney disease, and U.urealyticum which is more usually seen in urine samples, can be found in some types of bladder stones.

In men, about 15-20% of cases show U.urealyticum as a cause for non-gonococcal urethritis but research does not yet prove that it is the causative organism for prostatitis or urethritis, although thought possible. One would imagine that, since the male urinary tract follows through from the foreskin of the penis to the prostate gland, organisms encounter no particular barriers en route and that over time, incursive infection could well take place.

M.fermentans and M. penetrans have been isolated from HIV-sero-positive patients and discovered recently in blood, genital tract, and deep tissue samples from homosexuals, bisexuals and others with the condition. These two mycoplasmas are intensely opportunistic, colonising well in immuno-depressed victims.

The immune system becomes depressed for many reasons not just in HIV patients. Mercury amalgam poisoning may be the commonest cause of immuno-depression in society because of the fulsome use of it in the dental surgery. The constant drip of leaking mercury has to attract lymphocytes to try to control the poison. Many environmental toxins outside our control - such as fluoride in water and toothpastes, excessive electrical exposure from pylons, mobile phones, computers, chlorine in tap water and swimming pools, lead in car exhausts fumes, fungicides, pesticides and insecticides on foodstuffs - together with a host of other modern contributions keep our immune systems today overworked as never before in history. Serious life-threatening illnesses of all sorts will depress the immune system and, of course, we all know about stress, sleep deprivation and overwork.

Immuno-suppressive treatments such as steroids, chemotherapy and radiation have been seen to cause septicaemia by M.hominis. M.pneumoniae and U.uryliticum have been shown as a causative feature of septic arthritis. Mycobacteria are now becoming implicated in many forms of arthritis, bone and joint pain by knowledgable researchers but this is not yet filtering through to doctors.

TREATMENT

Finding the right antibiotic is difficult because mycoplasmas of all sorts fail to have affinities to the usual range. The culture Report should include antibiotics that have been tested against your specific bacteria, though the one most regularly used with best results is Doxycycline. According to how many months or years Mycoplasma or Ureaplasma has been inside your body somewhere, so the presiding physician should design the duration and strength of Doxycycline.

Hunner's Ulcer.

Emeritus Professor Guy L.R. Hunner was born in Wisconsin in 1868. He was passionate about becoming a doctor and obtained entrance to Johns Hopkins Medical School in Baltimore after college. He began working in the gynaecology department with Howard Kelly who had invented a technique for examining bladders with his own home-made cystoscope. Wanting to look further into the bladder, Kelly also devised a balloon that inflated bladders for more thorough inspection. Hunner became interested in the urological aspects of gynaecological investigations and was soon put in charge of this department.

In 1902, Hunner went into private practice in Baltimore but still helped out at Johns Hopkins when required. Using the balloon device, he discovered bladder ulcers in chronic cystitis giving his name to them. Hunner wrote a Paper on this ulcer that became his trademark:

'*Consideration on a new viewpoint on the aetiology of renal tuberculosis*', pub: American Journal of Obstetrics and Gynaecology, 1932, 24: 703-728.

It seems to have also been published in the American Journal of Obstetrics again in 1932, but shortened to 4 pages.

Kindly towards all sick people and animals, he frequently let the poor off paying bills both private and hospital often paying them himself. Patients would come to recuperate in his own home and so did sick animals! Haven't times moved on! Professor Hunner died in 1957.

As I write this piece, I have in front of me a large medical textbook entitled "Urology", Second Edition published by Blackwell Science and written/edited by two urologists in the UK called John Blandy and Christopher Fowler. So much in urological study is over-scientific and unreasonable especially when it comes to actually making the patient well. This textbook is reasonable and walking along the line that I have pondered for some years. It confirms what I stated at the beginning of this segment that IC is merely medical jargon and not some newfangled disease.

But is Hunner's Ulcer actually a bladder response to Myco and Ureaplasmas? Is this ulceration a continuing process from mere reddened patches on the bladder wall? Medical textbooks certainly neatly call them together as one and the same and many recent Papers on the web do likewise.

Hunner's Ulcer, in surgery, is diagnosed when the bladder under liquid distension starts to crack its surface and bleed. It is known as cascade bleeding. There are Mast cells present in biopsies as well as inflammatory cells. In searching with due diligence for TB of the bladder similar biopsies are performed and requests made to culture for M.tuberculosis if that is suspected from other lines of investigation.

Now I wonder whether similar research attempts to look for M.hominis or U.ureaplasma have been undertaken in cases of Hunner's Ulcer.

Scientific studies do not seem to have done such work on mycobacteria but concentrated on diseases such as lupus erythematous, scleroderma or autoimmune thyroiditis.

It should be time to conduct conclusive studies on Hunner's ulcer in relation to Mycobacteria, especially those of genital origin. I have found bladder biopsy samples containing Myco plasma.

CHAPTER THREE

3 The Real Cause

It is my contention from seeing and treating many patients that mycoplasmas and ureaplasmas are the result of some kind of sexual congress either oral or genital or both. In my opinion it commences from a dirty foreskin somewhere and this initial dirty foreskin infects countless vaginas and other penile skin during the course of a modern sexual lifestyle.

Undoubtedly, people have more sexual partners now because of contraception and abortion, the failure of marriage and faithfulness and increased travel 'opportunities'. Its no good being preachy simply because no-one takes any notice of it anyway, but I'm afraid its true!

DIAGNOSIS OF MYCOBACTERIA

I maintain that Interstititial Cystitis is not mere inflammation as Dr Gillespie states, nor is it enterococcal, as Dr Fugazzotto maintains since most labs ought to have found the old Strep fecalis with many still conventionally sampling and diagnosing it. But I do allow that a combination of poor patient sample preparation combined with poor laboratory knowledge may sort many so-called IC victims into this enterococcal category. It is still not correct to call this form of bacterial cystitis anything other than just that, bacterial cystitis. A plain bacterial cystitis is still not my idea of non-stop variable levels of pain twenty four hours a day seven days a week for many years.

All over the web are scientific papers and studies on IC. Just go to www.google.com and up come scores of studies and links. There are many projects in hand to try to break the puzzle but as yet no-one has made the sensible links that I have through my own, and other's, patients' histories. Specific lab cultures and in one case bladder biopsies, have shown our initial diagnosis of Mycobacteria or Ureaplasmas to be correct. Effective use of sensitive antibiotic treatment has won the day with every single IC patient fully recovered.

Cultures and Biopsies

Full blown so-called IC has horrendous impacts upon victims' lives and bladder biopsies taken from such victims usually show granulated or ulcerated patches which then apparently confirm to the presiding physycian that this is truly a verifiable case of IC. A biopsy is removal from any organ, in this case the bladder wall, a small piece of skin or tissue to be put later under a microscope. The microbiologist will then check for bacterial or fungal colonies, or anything else the surgeon specifically requests.

Whilst not every victim is biopsied at the ulcer stage it is perfectly possible to biopsy granulated, reddened bladder wall patches - IF the surgeon has any inkling of what he should be requesting a biopsy for!

To start with, the operation should be performed in a theatre within the same building as a laboratory bench able to culture mycoplasmas and ureaplasmas. The system and hospital should be known as efficient, i.e. some member of staff in the theatre will dedicate themself to walking your biopsy specimens straight into microbiology where it should go quickly into broth or onto a culture dish with the correct mediums for accurate organism enrichment and growth.

The surgeon or presiding nurse should have written "all bacteria, fungi, PLUS Mycoplasma and Ureaplasma" on the specimen container. Preferably the patient should double check that these are ready whilst being attended to in pre-anaesthetic. Ask to see the containers!!! If they do not say Mycoplasma and Ureaplasma, sit up and refuse the anaesthetic until you have either seen the marked containers or watched them now being marked in front of you!! Trust no-one!! You won't want to go through anaesthesia and recovery for six weeks again simply because some fool in theatre has 'forgotten' to do this or because the surgeon is behind schedule and can't be bothered!!

Also request at this time that plenty of painkillers are ready for you immediately surgery concludes, or back in the ward or your room. Having patches of bladder lining cut off is bound to be painful when you next urinate; it will also ache for a few days. To counteract this in addition to strong pain relief, drink plenty once nausea has gone, add some Mis pot cit, Cystopurin for UK patients, whatever else is offered in the States that you have found helpful in the past, perhaps something herbal or homeopathic like the marvellous Arnica. I'd suggest 3-4 pillules under the tongue as needed. Dilute urine does not sting, concentrated urine does. Bottle Wash as normal to keep new bacteria out of this even more tender bladder. It may take a month to six weeks still using occasional pain relief before effects of this surgery wear off and you become more comfortable.

Doxycycline

If the biopsies show positive for Myco or Ureaplasma start Doxycycline immediately at a long strong dose. Doxycyline usually comes out top of the list to stop these organisms reproducing. One of the patients I cared for, who travelled to see me from Houston, Texas, passed her first pain-free urine in twenty years after a ten day dose of 6 capsules a day. Her urine samples, vaginal swabs and a bladder biopsy all showed Ureaplasma uryliticum.

She had been in trouble for twenty years!! Twenty years!! and no-one in America had checked for the mycoplasmas or ureaplasmas! She had been wrongly told in the States that previous cystoscopies showed ulceration, we found none in London but there were plenty of granulated and reddened patches from which the urologist gathered six specimens. Either the ulcers had subsided which is unlikely, or she had been lied to so that the presiding physician could absolve himself from further responsibility and repeat visits. 'Take the money and see them out' is what I call this phenomenon! Most doctors are quick to point out that there is no cure and they wave a sad goodbye! A box of tissues is small comfort for 'negative' diagnoses.

All the patients I have ever counselled with so-called Interstitial Cystitis have been found to have a species of these two organisms, Mycoplasma or Ureaplasma, upon correct urine sampling and vaginal swabbing just because I suspected it from Case History and because the bacteriologist taking the samples requested the lab to culture specifically. The lab, which of course is capable of testing for Myco and Ureaplasmas, confirmed all the suspected diagnoses. **It is no good sending samples to a lab with no facility for testing these organisms.**

Dosage

In normal urinary tract infection the dose is minimal at five days of a single 100mg capsule. But ask the medical officer of the drug company what the maximum dose is and you will find that it can be taken for a month! Courses can be individually designed and it is best to hit a chronic infection with 6 capsules a day for 7-10 days. This is called the Venereal Disease dose and truthfully if the victim has been suffering for anything over a couple of months, this is worth contemplating because M.homini and U.urealyticum are tough bastards to shift. They reproduce cyclically and when you think the twinges have gone, they return a week or so later. Each repeat course is likely to meet with the same response, so take a longer steady dose and you beat the cycle. Most antibotics are bacteriostatic, not bactericidal so they cause mycoplasmas and urea uryliticum to merely 'march on the spot until all reproduction ceases rather than be killed outright. They need to be stopped from reproducing and eventually there are none left either reproducing or marching!

Doxycycline can cause nausea unless you take it with meals, because it is not an easy antibiotic to digest. Referring back to my own three year brush with M.hominis, I took 4 capsules a day for four days and the discharge never returned, but I do know of women whose doctors just prescribed five days of 1 capsule and they needed two or three more courses. Treatment should most definitely be personally designed within the drug company's accepted range and should attempt to hit mycoplasmas and urea uryliticum hard and fast.

For such seriously infected victims, relief at a positive bacterial outcome from the lab report is enormous, absolutely enormous.

My own best guesses at dosage are:

- under six months suffering:
  3 x100mg capsules per day for five days
- under five years suffering:
  4x100mg capsules per day for six days or longer if twinges remain
- under ten years suffering:
  5 x 100mg capsules per day for six days or longer if twinges persist
- over ten years suffering:
  6 x 100mg capsules per day for 8-10 days, no longer, and unnecessary!!

BUT here is where recovery begins from years of pain and distress. Passing pain-free urine and knowing what caused all this is a huge relief. You were not crazy, it was not all in the mind, it **was** a real live organism, or to be correct, colonies of them that have been responsible for ruining your life. Use the courts if you have the energy and inclination, go on the TV, write to the magazines and newspapers, get it out on the web through the IC sites, anything at all to stop the ignorance and suffering of others both lay and medical. Such channelled revenge will also aid your mental recovery because mental recovery as well as physical will be needed.

Your sexual partner MUST also take a high dose otherwise there will simply be a re-infection. If his foreskin is heavy and practically unwashable think about circumcision because repeat episodes between you will eventually stop Doxycycline from working. Re-infection also leaves permanent miniscule scars into which bacteria gain easier entry each time to kidneys, bladder or urethra.

Recovery

There follows not only the convalescence from surgery for about six weeks but also the recovery from such stringent antibiotics. **The bladder physically needs to rest;** it needs very loving care and thoughtfulness. The immune system needs masses of mineral and vitamin supplements. Anti-fungal drugs, both oral and local, will be needed to counteract the loss of natural gut bacterial/ fungal competition. Perhaps a nutritionist will advise herbal, naturopathic, homeopathic preparations to stimulate immune recovery from all the drugs, anaesthetic and depression.

Conclusion

This third book of the Encyclopaedia is about long term, ongoing, chronic pain, frequency, malaise and distress. Of all the offerings in here I maintain that the first line of investigation is certainly MycoUreaplasma. It has come up in samples from every one of my so-called IC patients who have previously been everywhere and done everything to no avail.

No patient seeing me has had so-called enterococcus infections because their urine sample results, which I always want copies of, have at least in UK been found to have Streptococcus fecalis if it is there and which was the old name for this infection. Perhaps the patient is at fault because no personality like myself exists in America, either in media pieces or in literature, to bang the gong for informed and careful patient sample-taking or perhaps lab methodology differs.

In Summary

Find the nearest lab which tests for Mycobacteria, find the doctor, take the sample correctly, wait for the diagnosis, take Doxycycline appropriately. I think if all my information is followed to the letter, it will be found that IC, even with ulcers and granulation, is due to Myco Ureaplasma of the main genital group and that careful sexual hygiene by bottle washing will prevent repeat trouble. Oral and genital sex are the commonest contributing factors and changing sexual partners is very risky indeed.

Your life quality may be determined by an unclean and bacterially contaminated foreskin. Using a condom only before ejaculation is no protection whatsoever because oral sex and initial penetration may have done the damage already. The amount of distress caused by unsolved chronic bladder infection is so great that I want to see a return to male circumcision.

Total chastity is a thing of the past and I am realistic, but at no time should you contemplate one-night stands drunk or not drunk. Give friendship a chance first then talk sex through before bed beckons more strongly. If any symptoms start sort yourself out using this book and all its wonderful advice.

Educate your doctor, too and become one of my millions of disciples. You are not alone but one of millions of women who throughout all past, present and future ages will start cystitis at some time in life. Be absolutely inquisitive, resolute and intelligent about searching for the cause or causes because no doctor has sufficient time or knowledge to do it for you. Use the medical profession when you want a specific test but don't let them operate unnecessarily or kid you into unproductive cystoscopies or dilations.

You must take charge yourself and armed with the knowledge from this book, sort yourself out!

APPENDIX

Glossary of Terms

Anaemia low level of iron in the blood

Anus opening for passage of feces

Artery blood vessel carrying blood from the heart

Bacteria germs

Bicarbonate of soda baking soda, an alkalizing agent

Bladder elastic sac in the pelvic region which stores urine

Candida thrush; a fungus infection of the mouth, vagina and rectum

Catheterization insertion of a small tube to withdraw urine from the bladder

Cauterization burning away of infected skin

Cervicitis any inflammation of the cervix

Cervix neck of the womb

Colitis inflammation of the colon (part of the bowel)

Cystoscopy an operation for investigation of the bladder

Diabetes illness caused by lack of insulin in the bloodstream

Dialysis artificial cleansing of the blood by a machine

Dilatation/dilation enlargement of cervix or urethra by the insertion of rods

Distal urethral stenosis condition of the bladder during menopause or old age

Diuretic an agent which stimulates the production of urine

Diverticulitis inflammation of the bowel

Diverticulum small false bladder growth

E. Coli natural bacteria which inhabit the bowel

Enuresis bed wetting

Episiotomy an operation on the perineum during difficult childbirth

Epithelium skin

Estrogen hormone involved in ovulation

Foreskin skin covering the end of the penis

Fungus growth of detrimental yeast organisms

Gonadotrophin hormone involved in ovulation

Hexachlorophine an antiseptic used frequently in hospitals

Hormone a chemical messenger carrying instructions from glands to organs

Hormone imbalance incorrect balance of hormones

Hysterectomy removal of all or part of the internal female sexual organs

IVP intravenous pyelogram, or kidney X-ray

Labia (majoralminora) folds of skin which protect urethral and vaginal orifices

Litmus paper chemical papers able to test for acidity/alkalinity

MSU mid-stream urine specimen

Menopause natural process involving termination of menstruation

Micturition act of passing urine

Micturating cystogram an X-ray taken during urination

Monilia thrush; a fungus infection of the mouth, rectum and vagina

Ovulation release of unfertilized female egg from the ovaries

Perineum base of the body's trunk containing excretory orifices

Pituitary gland chief sexual gland of the brain responsible for most hormone activity

Potassium citrate alkalizing agent

Prostate gland male sexual gland through which passes the urethra

Pyelitis kidney disease

Radiographer specialist in X-ray techniques

Rectum tube for passing of stools to the outside

Reflux urine flow in the wrong direction

Renal scarring scarring of the kidney by constant disease

Sphincter valve valve attached to the sphincter muscles controlling output of urine

Streptococcus a form of bacteria

Trichomonas sexually transmitted disease

Ureters tubes carrying urine from the kidneys to the bladder

Urethra tube carrying urine from the bladder

Urethral syndrome medically unaccountable symptoms of cystitis without bacteria

Urologist doctor specializing in renal organs

Uterus womb

Vagina birth canal

Vaginal thrush milky, irritative discharge from the vagina

Vaginitis any inflammation of the vagina

Vein blood vessel carrying blood to the heart

Yeast a fungus invasion of tissue, local or systemic